Scientific Training for
Triathletes

Philip F. Skiba, D.O., M.S.

Dedication

This work is dedicated to all of the scientists and physicians who gave of themselves in my education and training, and to all those who seek to improve themseleves through the knowledge I hope to pass on.

Copyright © 2004 by Philip Friere Skiba, D.O., M.S.
United States Copyright Number: TXu1-199-683

All rights reserved. Except for use in a review, reproduction or utilization of this work in any form or by any electronic, mechanical means, now known or hereafter invented is forbidden without the written permission of the author.

Printed in the United States of America.

Philip Friere Skiba
philip.skiba@att.net
www.PhysFarm.com

Design and layout by Kathryn Skiba

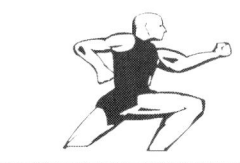

TABLE OF CONTENTS

Preface		v
CHAPTER 1	Back to Basics	9
CHAPTER 2	How Do I Figure Out My Own Physiologic Parameters	21
CHAPTER 3	What Kinds of Workouts Train Which Energy System	27
CHAPTER 4	The Underlying Principle of Training: Specificity	49
CHAPTER 5	Strength Training	53
CHAPTER 6	Detraining: What Happens When We Get Hurt, or Lazy	57
CHAPTER 7	Periodization: The Reductionist Viewpoint	61
CHAPTER 8	Feeding the Machine	69
CHAPTER 9	Tapering To Race	89
CHAPTER 10	Race Day	95
CHAPTER 11	Aid By Technology	103
Epilogue		115
Post Script		117
Works Cited		119
About the Author		127

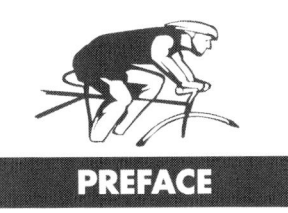

PREFACE

As a physician and triathlon coach, I hear the same questions over and over from my patients and clients. "What is VO₂max?"; "How do I increase my lactate threshold?"; "Will this supplement or accessory make me faster?"; "What should my strategy be?" There is much information available explaining the physiology of exercise. Unfortunately, much of it is inaccessible to the average athlete who does not have a strong background in the sciences. Thus, many athletes turn to the Internet for advice. The Internet is a great resource, however, much advice dispensed there is either coaching lore, opinion, marketing hype, or consists of questionable factoids dispensed by people with still more questionable credentials. It is difficult for the average person to know who is interested in educating them and who is attempting to sell their own particular brand of hair tonic, so to speak.

I wrote this manual with the express intent of educating athletes who are either self-coaching, or perhaps have a coach but want to understand their workout schedule. It will also be of use to the coach with much 'practical knowledge,' but little scientific knowledge of how the body responds to exercise. However, this manual has little to do with the actual act of coaching of endurance athletes. You won't find any detailed training plans or workout schedules in these pages. As exercise physiologist Dr. Andrew Coggan once wrote, "Coaching is not a science, but all coaching should be based on scientific principles." My hope is that by the time you finish this book, you will be able to design workout protocols consistent with what is known of exercise physiology. Moreover, you will be able to identify whether a particular workout, supplement, or strategy is sensible in light of what we know of science.

I do not presume to cover all that is known about exercise physiology and related fields in these few pages. This work is not meant to be exhaustive: it is a starting point for your athletic education. It is a means to get you training efficiently and more importantly, safely and without gimmicks. Before now, athletes were largely required to sift through the many coaching manuals on the market, which often contradict each other (and sometimes, themselves), in order to pull out pearls of wisdom. If the athlete had questions or was interested in understanding the basis of certain information, he or she had the daunting task of seeing out someone educated on the subject, or proceeding to the nearest university library. In these pages, I have done the legwork for you. I have attempted to digest the latest scientific and medical information so that you can use it to achieve your best.

In these pages you will note that I have included many references, so that should you wish to read the primary literature directly, you may do so. I have done this because you should not have to simply "take my word for it" because I have some letters after my name. If you find some information here that you feel is questionable, I have made it possible for you to track down the primary source of the information so that you can decide for yourself. In fact, I encourage this sort of thing. You are your own best teacher, and moreover, you may find that you have a particular interest in the subject and some unique insight which other authors have not discovered. A good starting point might be for you to purchase a copy of an exercise physiology text as a reference (Astrand's *Textbook of Work Physiology*, for example), should you be interested in further reading or explanation.

I often hear the comment, "Everyone has different advice, and every athlete is different. JFT (Just Freaking Train)." I agree with the former, but could not disagree more with the latter. Medically and physiologically speaking, each of us is different. It is important that we remember that each of us has individual strengths and weaknesses. We may find we have exceptional powers of healing and recovery, or patterns of injury we wish to alter. However, at the most basic level, each of us is governed by simple (and not-so-simple) biologic truths. While they do not tell the entire story, we would well heed them as a gross outline to direct training if we wish to see the best results possible. Your goal, or that of your coach, is to critically evaluate your strengths and weaknesses and adapt the studied techniques you will find here to your particular physiology. You need to specifically direct your efforts to your particular situation to obtain the best results.

Finally, this work covers the more practical issues of equipment selection and use, which have been the subject of much scientific study. These points can at the minimum serve to make your sporting life significantly easier and at the highest level will make the difference between winning and being just another competitor. Hopefully, this will assist you in critically evaluating what is on the market and making sense of the often outrageous claims manufacturers make. You are being bombarded with advertisements from the moment you open a magazine or walk into a bicycle shop. When you turn on the Olympics, swimsuit manufacturers are hoping you will see the latest racing getup and drop a few hundred bucks because you absolutely have to have it. I would like you to be making an informed choice.

What this manual will not do is turn you into the next Lance Armstrong, Peter Reid or Paula Radcliffe. The most elite of the elite athletes have a genetic gift for athletics that they are able to maximize through smart training. Hopefully, reading this will help you to enjoy the sports you compete in more fully, and perhaps help you lift your performance to the next level. I firmly believe that the biggest factor in your performance and health is you. Only you can listen to your body and say, "I feel great today, maybe I can put in a little extra work." Or, "My knee pain is getting worse. I ought to see my doctor." Above all, you need to train smart. The most important organ to your performance is your brain. I want to help you use it.

The Other Dr. Phil

CHAPTER 1

Back to Basics

I f you read any of the cycling, triathlon, or running books or magazines on the market today, you are likely to find terms like VO$_2$, Lactate Threshold, and efficiency thrown around. Do you know what any of them mean? You might not if you don't have a background in exercise science or medicine. Don't feel bad: many of the people spouting abbreviations and numbers at you don't know either. To make matters more confusing, there are a number of authors and coaches who are inventing new terms to describe ideas that already have an associated scientific term. I am not entirely sure why this is. Perhaps they feel they need their own jargon to set their particular training program apart from the rest, or perhaps they are simply ignorant of the appropriate language which is accepted in the field of exercise science. I have no doubt they mean well, but it sure can get confusing.

Before we can get to the nitty-gritty of things like the lactate threshold or VO$_2$max, we need to get on the same page in terms of the very basic workings of your body. In order to make the energy you need to exercise (or even to just remain alive), your body processes fat and carbohydrate (sugar) with oxygen. Your cells don't just run on one fuel or the other, they must first turn it into a kind of universal chemical energy your cells can use to do the things they need to do (contract, build hormones, conduct electrical signals, etc.) called adenosine triphosphate (ATP). You can think of it in terms of your car: you need to process crude oil to make the refined gasoline that makes your engine run. Your body stores these types of fuel as either fat in adipose cells or glycogen (the storage form of sugar) in your muscle cells and in your liver.

Your muscle cells use both fat and carbohydrates for fuel. The fuel balance is determined by how hard and/or long you are exercising (figure 1.0). If you are exercising slowly, you are burning more fat and less carbohydrate; the reverse is true if you are exercising very quickly. Interestingly, you actually have different types of muscle cells, each of which has a particular fuel preference for the work they do. There are essentially 3 types, which are called Type I (slow twitch oxidative), Type IIx (fast twitch glycolytic) and Type IIa (fast oxidative glycolytic).

The type I cells are the ones we are most interested in training for endurance exercise. They burn mostly fat and have oxidative enzymes to do this, so we call them oxidative, but are somewhat weaker than the other 2 types. However, they are extremely resistant to fatigue. They are also referred to as "slow twitch," meaning that they do not fire as quickly as the type II cells. The type IIx cells are fast twitch. They fire much more quickly, and are much stronger, but tire more quickly. They also recover quickly. They burn much more sugar than they do fat, so we call them glycolytic. Type IIa are what is called "fast oxidative glycolytic." In other words, you can train them to go either way. If you wanted to

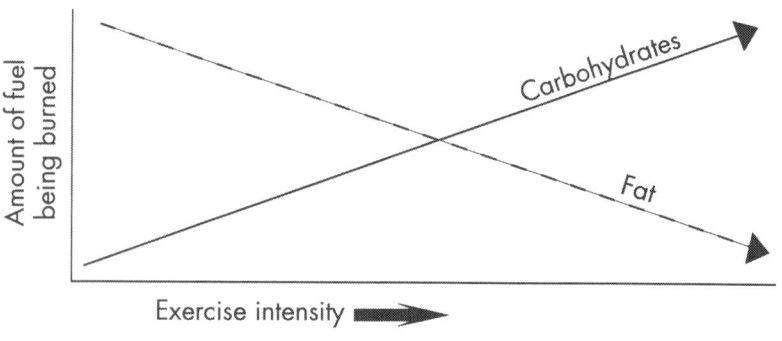

Figure 1.0   The relationship between fuel type and exercise intensity.

sprint, you could train them to be more like the fast twitch guys. If you wanted to jog, you could train them to be more like the slow twitch guys.

You recruit these different cells based on activity, as I alluded to above. Think of it this way: you have ten cases of beer you are taking up a flight of stairs to a party. You have a choice: try and lug them all up at once, or do one at a time. If you take one up at a time, you will be mostly using your slow twitch fibers. You've got a lot of work to do, so you recruit a bunch of weaker fibers who won't get tired easily. If you try to carry them up at once, you are doing more of a "maximal effort," so you recruit all the really strong fast twitch cells in addition to all the weaker ones, because you need as much help as you can get. However, you should note that activities are rarely "easy" or "maximal." Also, even doing easier tasks, you will start recruiting the stronger cells as the weaker ones get tired.

Earlier, we said that you need to process fuel with oxygen to get energy. It is somewhat difficult to directly measure your overall energy output, but it is relatively easy to figure out how much oxygen you are using with a gas analyzer. Thus, we often describe the intensity of exercise in terms of how much oxygen you are using, or your oxygen uptake. VO_2 is defined as the volume of oxygen, in milliliters per minute that your body is using at any

> **Three Kinds of Muscle Cells**
>
> **Slow twitch cells:**
> - used mostly in endurance exercise
> - extremely resistant to fatigue
> - burn mostly fat
>
> **Fast twitch cells:**
> - fire much more quickly
> - stronger than slow twitch cells
> - recover quickly
> - burn much more sugar than fat
>
> **Fast oxidative gycolytic cells:**
> - can be trained to have either slow twitch or fast twitch characteristics

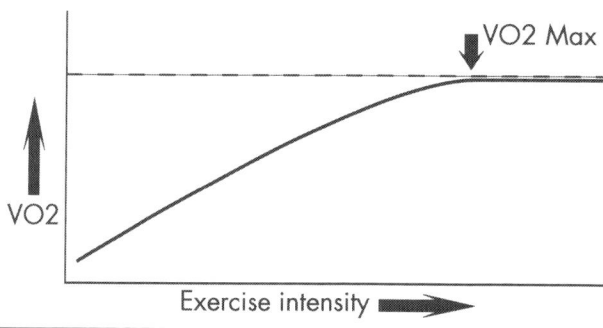

Figure 1.1 Relationship between oxygen uptake and exercise intensity.

given moment. For example, if you are sitting quietly, your oxygen uptake is very low. If you are running a 5k, your oxygen uptake is high. VO₂max is the maximum amount of oxygen you are able to use during maximal or exhaustive exercise.[1] It is a very good indicator of your maximal endurance athletic performance. However, the person with the highest number is not always the winner. There are other factors at work. We will discuss them later.

You will often see the VO₂ number corrected for body weight. In other words, if you weigh 50 kg and I weigh 100kg (1 kilogram= about 2.2 lbs), but each of us has a VO₂max of 5000 ml/min, we can compare ourselves by saying that yours is 100 ml per kilogram per minute, and mine is 50 ml per kg per min. This is what really matters in weight bearing activities[2] or in uphill cycling: how high it is in relation to your size/weight. Think of it this way: a Ferrari and a big truck might have the same horsepower, but the Ferrari goes uphill faster because it weighs less. In other words, it has a higher power to weight ratio (figure 1.2).

If we measured your maximal oxygen uptake in all three sports, we would likely find different values in each. This does not mean that your VO₂max itself changes. You may not be a good enough athlete in all three sports to be able to drive your body to that limit. What you will achieve in each is called VO₂ peak. You may not be trained enough to reach a VO₂max in any sport at all. However, with training, you would probably be able to hit a maximal value, that is, a value determined by the limit of your heart, and not the limits of the rest of your body, in your main sport. In other words, if you are a career runner, you can probably drive yourself to the VO2max limit while running, but maybe not while cycling or swimming. It is an academic point, but one worth making. VO2max is the *ulitmate* limit, determined by how much blood your heart can get to your exercising muscles. VO2 peak is your functional limit, meaning it is the best you can do given your current training and ability level.

A helpful way of expressing VO2 is as a percentage of maximum VO2. We do this because we want to divide our training program into levels of intensity, and we want to be able to talk about them to each other and make sense. For example, (and I am just making these numbers up) you and I might both do a workout at an oxygen uptake of 40 ml/kg/min. However, if each of us has a different maximum, those might be very different workouts. If my maximum is 80, then I had an easy workout, but if yours is 50, you were going quite hard. Now, if you tell me you were working at 80% percent of your maximum, and I tell you I was working at 50% of mine, that makes more sense.

"Okay," You are asking, "But how do I find out what my VO2max (or peak) is?" Well, that is complicated. The real way to do it is take you to a laboratory, give you a mouthpiece that is hooked up to some hoses, and measure how much oxygen you breathe in and how much carbon dioxide you breathe out at rest. Then, we run you on a treadmill, faster and faster until you just

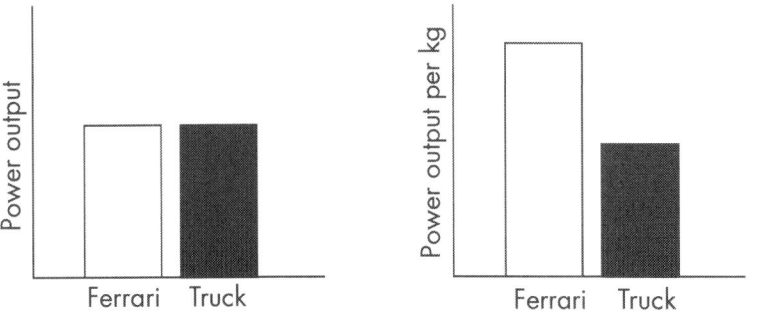

Figure 1.2   The concept of power to weight ratio.

about collapse, all the while making the same measurements. The good news is that the absolute number isn't all that important, and we can actually make a pretty good guesstimate using less tortuous methodology. We will discuss this further later.

Again, VO_2 is a measure of how fit your cardiovascular system is. It is primarily determined by how much oxygen rich blood your heart can deliver to your working muscles. Your muscles, once well trained, will use as much oxygen as your heart can provide. Thus, a higher VO_2 is better. The good news is that you can train in certain ways to increase your VO_2. The bad news is that those changes become more and more difficult to realize as you get more fit. (Realize, however, that the further, small changes you might realize will prove important, especially at the highest level of competition where races are won and lost by small margins). Finally, there is more good news: earlier, we learned that what really mattered was your VO_2 per amount of body weight. Well, that means that if you lose weight, your VO_2max *must* go up, and thus you will get faster because your muscles have less total weight to move around.

> **VO_2 is a measure of how fit your cardiovascular system is.**

Another facet worth mentioning is the idea of the slow component of VO_2. There has been a significant amount of work showing that once you pass a certain level of intensity (the lactate threshold), oxygen consumption begins to increase slowly upward, even if your work load isn't. There are a number of reasons this may be, and we will discuss them later, because it turns out that there are more important issues to your exercise performance than raw VO_2.

The next topic for discussion is the lactate threshold. Before we discuss the threshold, let's consider the lactate. Lactate is one of the products of carbohydrate metabolism in your muscles. When your muscles are working at a reasonable level, you do not have much net accumulation of lactate, because you are mostly using fat for fuel. However, as the workload rises to a level that you are not well-trained enough to meet with relatively more fat burning and relatively less carbohydrate burning, your fuel balance shifts toward carbohydrates and more lactate begins to be produced. To some extent, lactate is taken up and broken down by your body. However, you will eventually exercise hard enough that production outstrips elimination. When this begins to occur, lactate builds up in your circulation and muscles.

> **Lactate threshold** is scientifically defined as a rise in lactate of 1 millimole (mmol) per liter over your exercise baseline.

Lactate threshold is scientifically defined as a rise in lactate of 1 millimole (mmol) per liter over your exercise baseline (figure 1.3). In other words, if we put you on a hamster wheel and made you run faster and faster, we would initially see a constant level of lactate. You would eventually get to a workload that caused the lactate in your blood to bump up by the above amount. It would climb higher and higher if we kept increasing the work, until such a time as you could not continue and you fell over gasping, spinning around and around like a cat in a clothes dryer.

There are other terms used by authors in the field such as Mean Lactate Steady State (MLSS), or Onset of Blood Lactate Accumulation (OBLA) (about 4 mmol/liter of lactate). There are advantages and disadvantages to these terms. For example, an advantage of the terms OBLA or MLSS is that they seem to be

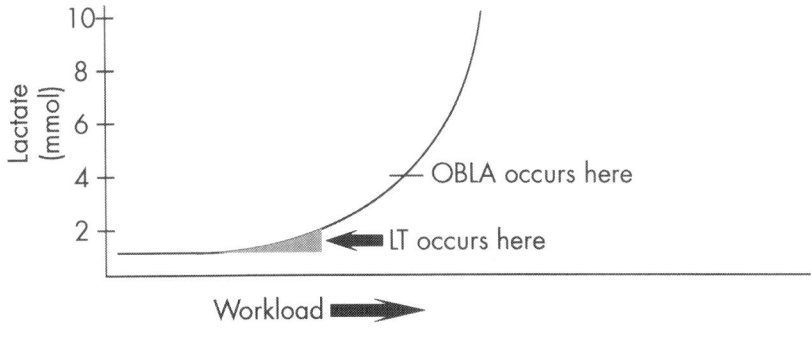

Figure 1.3   Relationship between lactate and workload.

better correlated with the pace athletes and coaches seem to consider "threshold pace."[3] They also seem better correlated with the idea most athletes have of the workings of lactate, in other words, since MLSS is the highest work level attainable without a continual increase in lactate, they consider this their true "threshold."[18] The disadvantage is that these things occur *after* the lactate has begun to rise. The cow is already out of the barn at this point, so to speak. Another disadvantage is that no one specific number would work for everyone.

Is there a real difference between training at LT and training at OBLA/MLSS? To be honest, I don't know. Speed at OBLA/MLSS is higher than it is at LT. My opinion is that both are training the same mechanism and there will not be a huge difference between the two, though you need to be careful with excessive "threshold running" as it can wear you out. My experience is that athletes overall feel better, but also sometimes feel they are not training "hard enough" when they are working at a true LT pace. However, they are able to put in more time at LT than they can at OBLS/MLSS/ "threshold pace". It also seems to me (and this is supported by some authors, as we will see in the next section) that as athletes become better trained, they need a more severe training stimulus to realize additional gains.

Finally, some people refer to the LT as the anaerobic threshold; anaerobic meaning "not aerobic," which is an absolute misnomer since you are, in fact, still using oxygen. This is a long-standing misunderstanding and I feel we must correct it. LT is *not* due to some inability to deliver oxygen to your muscles. Again, lactate threshold is the result of a metabolic change; in other words, the fuel shift from predominantly fat to a higher percentage of carbohydrate.

It is important for you to realize a couple of things. Firstly, the above is really a simplification of the lactate story. We can go on for quite some time about why and how the lactate begins to rise, and the exact mechanism of its uptake and processing by other cells in the body. Indeed, people much smarter than me have been putting this to committee for a long time. Rather than trying to put too fine a point on it, I think the best way for me to convey the meaning of the lactate threshold is as follows: the lactate threshold is the *effect of*, not the *cause of* your endurance capacity at any given time. What I mean is that around the time that the lactate starts creeping up, there are *lots* of other changes going on in your body. You are recruiting more type II (fast twitch) muscle fibers, your rate of breathing is going up, and your muscles are starting to use proportionally more glycogen, and proportionally less fat for fuel. Lactate is simply an easy way of monitoring a whole bunch of changes in your body. It is a way of looking at the "big picture." The object of training, at the end of the day, is to enable you to do more work before the lactate begins to rise in your blood; not because of the lactate per se, but because that means your body is overall more fit.

Your lactate threshold is probably more important to your triathlon performance than your raw VO_2, and moreover you can improve the amount of work you do at LT over a much longer period of time than we can your VO_2. As we said above, with specific training, your VO_2 starts to level off after a few months. Your work level at LT can be improved over a period of several years.

So how do we correlate LT with VO_2? We can inter-relate your VO_2 and LT by expressing your LT as a percentage of your VO_2. Recall that your work level at VO_2max is the highest level of work your cardiovascular system is capable of supporting for any significant length of time. Before you are well trained, your muscles cannot support that level of exercise for very long. On the other hand, you can exercise for quite some time around or below your lactate threshold. As we improve the function of your muscle with training, we raise the amount of work they can do at lactate threshold closer to the amount they can do at VO_2max. We might say that your LT occurs at 70% of your VO_2max. With training, you will be able to raise that percentage so that your LT occurs at 80% of your VO_2 (figure 1.4). In other words, you will overall be able to exercise faster and longer before lactate begins to accumu-

18 | CHAPTER 1
Back to Basics

late. You will be able to exercise longer at a workload closer to the maximum your body is capable of.

Now we come to endurance, and endurance means just that: your body's capacity to endure what you are putting it through, or how long it can carry on working. It is related to the workload you are subjecting your body to. For instance, you would obviously be able to exercise longer if you were walking than if you were running quite fast. Well, by training the first two you are also training your endurance capacity, that is, your ability to exercise longer. In fact, training at or near lactate threshold is probably going to give you the most bang for your buck in terms of time spent training and the results you see for

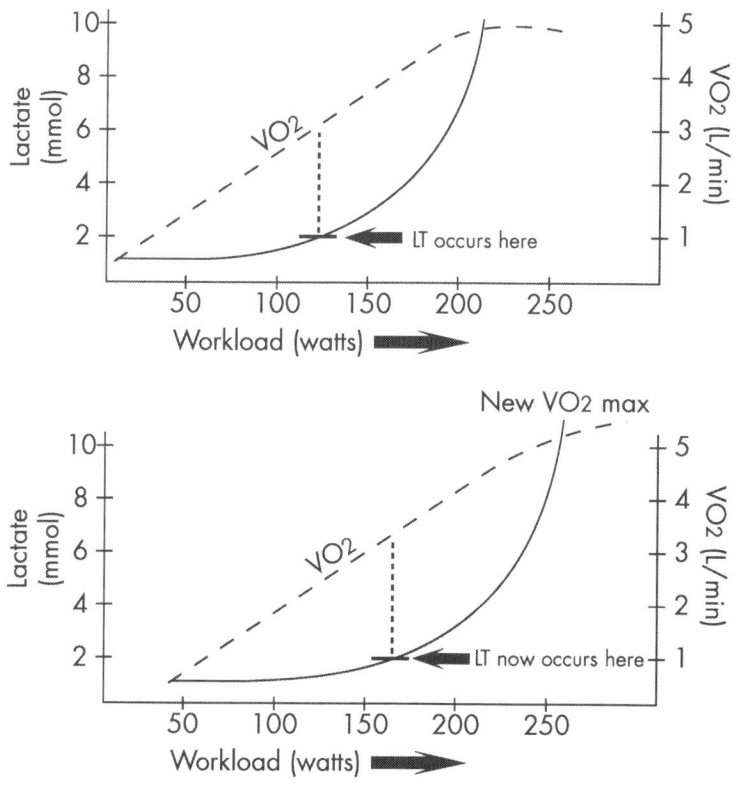

Figure 1.4 A & B   Relationship between lactate, oxygen uptake, and workload. Note the change between A (untrained) and B (trained).

that training in an increased endurance capacity. However, it can be difficult to train at that intensity constantly, so you will certainly have purely "endurance workouts." We will discuss these in the next chapter.

The last concept we will discuss is that of efficiency/economy. Essentially, you can consider this the minimization of cost while maximizing work done. For example, if you can hold a very streamlined position while swimming, more of your effort goes into pushing you forward and less goes into fighting the resistance of the water. Efficiency is something that is both learned and trained. You may learn how to swim more efficiently, but you train yourself to be efficient by practicing what you have learned until it becomes automatic. Presumably, you can refine your swim stroke throughout your life. Perfect practice makes perfect.

It is important to realize that scientists will use two different terms, efficiency and economy, when referring to different exercises. We don't need to split hairs quite so much, but we should talk about the difference. *Efficiency* is a term we borrow from our engineer friends. It is the ratio of work done to the amount of energy required to do that work. Efficiency is the term used in the cycling literature because it is easy to throw a power meter on a bike and measure the actual energy output and work done.

In the swimming and running literature, we refer to *economy*. It is the same idea, but since it is hard to wire a power meter to a person, we simply measure the amount of oxygen they use and compare it to how fast they go using that much oxygen. If two runners or swimmers of like size are tested, and they both go the same speed, the one using the less oxygen would be the more economical (figure 1.5). Looking at cyclists, if two similar cyclists are producing the same wattage, the one doing it with less oxygen is the more efficient. It is a fine point, but is one worth making.

20 | CHAPTER 1
Back to Basics

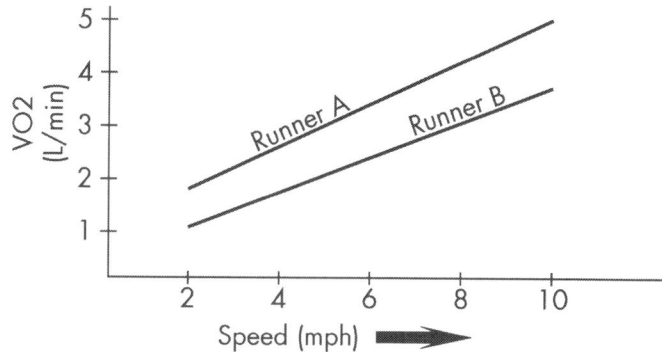

Figure 1.5 The concept of economy. If two runners of like size use different amounts of oxygen when running at the same speed, the one using less oxygen is said to be more economical. Thus, Runner B is more economical than Runner A.

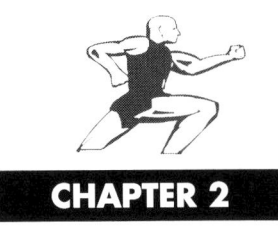

CHAPTER 2

How Do I Figure Out My Own Physiologic Parameters?

Now that I have told you all about what kinds of physiologic parameters we are interested in, we have a new problem. We need to figure out what your particular parameters are before we start training to change them. Or do we?

There are a number of ways of measuring your physiologic parameters. You can call up the physiology department of your local university, or other reputable place to get your testing done. They will put you on a treadmill, a stationary bike, and perhaps even a flume pool (hopefully, all three because each sport is going to give you different values), hook you up to a bunch of hoses, measure the gasses you inhale and exhale as they exercise the heck out of you and give you your numbers. They will tell you what pace and/or power output elicited what percentage of your VO₂max/VO₂peak.

The next step will be lactate threshold testing, where they will again work you in all three disciplines, constantly increasing the work and drawing blood by finger stick or by IV to make a lactate curve. They will identify your lactate threshold and tell you what pace/workload it occurs at in each sport.

With this information, you will be able to look at the table 3.0, or other reference and decide which paces/power outputs/percentages of your VO₂max you should be working at to maximize the training adaptations you want. You will purchase a power meter for your bike, so that you will always know precisely how hard you are working. You will do your threshold and interval run workouts on a measured course with a watch, or a GPS or other pacing tool so that you know you are working at just the right level. You will religiously watch the pace clock when you are in the pool so that you know you are hitting your times. Finally, you will buy a heart rate monitor, and correlate your heart rate to your workload at each level, so that you will know you are in the right ballpark if you have a hard time telling otherwise.

All of this testing may be somewhat expensive, which may or may not be important to you based on your financial means. It is about as "scientific" as you can get, and that is what this manual is supposed to be all about. However, I only recommend that approach for competitive athletes. I don't mean that only in terms of athletes going for the win, rather, you may be particularly competitive because you are trying to get every last ounce of performance out of yourself, even if you never take a win. I believe there is something honorable and noble in that. You should realize, however, that you might spend some money and not see an enormous performance increase per dollar.

Strictly speaking, I do not believe it is necessary to spend vast sums of money to determine your parameters, nor do I believe that the above extensive testing regimen is the only way to athletic success. Consider that Dr. Roger Bannister ran the first sub-4 minute mile without any such technology. He simply spent some of his daily workout running sub-minute quarter-mile intervals. A half-century later, with all the technology in the world, most of us will never match that feat. However, with a minimal investment in technology, we can make our sporting lives easier by getting more benefit from the amount of training time we have.

A good first investment is in a heart rate monitor; even an inexpensive one will do. There are many, many training programs out there which rely solely on the premise of using heart rate to determine workload. This works to some extent, but there are certain caveats which you must be aware of. First, is it a useable way of measuring intensity accurately? Yes, however, it is in general useful for monitoring "steady efforts." In other words, if you go

CHAPTER 2
How Do I Figure Out My Own Physiologic Parameters?

out for a workout that involves you exercising at a consistent pace for many minutes at a time, your heart rate will in general be proportional to your VO_2. However, heart rate is a very poor way of measuring short, intense efforts. This is because heart rate lags effort by some time. For example, if you get out of your chair and run up a flight of stairs, you will find that you feel your heart start hammering as or after you reach the top. In other words, your heart rate does not accurately reflect what you are doing right now. It is a little behind you.

> **Heart Rate Monitoring** is useful for monitoring steady efforts for many minutes at a time.

Another problem with heart rate as an indicator is that it is sensitive to many factors. For example, if you were a little dehydrated, you would find that your heart rate was higher at a given workload/pace that it typically was. When you are sleep deprived, your heart rate will be higher than usual. If you were ill, you would find the same thing. Also, certain medications can affect your heart rate. These factors are also useful to some extent in that they can help you monitor your overall training/health picture. You just need to remember that in absolute terms, it is unwise to rely on your heart rate as the sole measure of your effort.

For those of you who are just getting your feet wet in triathlon, I recommend a "holistic approach" to initially determine your training parameters. I recommend you learn to listen to your body, which when coupled with a few fun facts of physiology, and the aforementioned heart rate monitor can get you into the ballpark you need to be training in. You do not need to be a slave to it, but it will help you if you are like me, and have a hard time measuring your effort by feel alone. With this in mind, let us go on to:

How Do I Figure Out My VO₂max Without a Lab test?

My first question is, "Do you really need to know it?" What I mean by that is the following: the absolute number is not really important, unless you are interested in bragging to your friends. In terms of your training, what is important is knowing that you are exercising *at* or *near* it. From innumerable studies, we know that the VO_2max occurs for most healthy people within maybe 10-15 beats of their maximal heart rate. In fact, it may often occur at a lower workload or heart rate; however, if you can get within 10 beats of the maximum you are probably there. So, workouts aimed at improving this will need to take place to some extent at that level of intensity. We will get more into the specifics in the next chapter.

If you are *really* interested in knowing the number without an actual lab test, you can guesstimate your VO_2max by using a number of different nomograms available on the internet. These generally require your age and other vital charachteristics, and are not very accurate. There are other nomograms which will utilize your speed over a particular distance (for example, a 5k) to estimate VO_2max. These tend to be more accurate. Dr. Jack Daniels authored a paper on the subject some time ago, and his method and charts are available in his book *Daniels' Running Formula,* which is quite user friendly. This work has the added benefit of providing sound

---

Fun Activity #1:

Figure out your vVO2max for running.

1. Run on a track (or with a GPS receiver) at a speed of 8.5 km/hr.
2. Accelerate by 1 km/hr every 2 minutes.
3. The fastest speed you can hold for the entire 2 minutes without slowing down is your vVO2max.

Adapted from: Leger and Boucher. An indirect running multistage field test, the Universite de Montreal Track Test. Can J Appl Sports Sci; 5: 77-84. 1980.

Fun Activity #2:

Figure out your vVO2max/ pVO2max for cycling.

1. Ride on a quiet road on a day with little wind at an easy pace, or on a trainer with a power meter.
2. Accelerate by 1 km/hr every 2 minutes (or 10 watts every 2 minutes).
3. The fastest speed (or power) you can hold for the entire 2 minutes without slowing down is your vVO2max.

Adapted from: Leger and Boucher. An indirect running multistage field test, the Universite de Montreal Track Test. Can J Appl Sports Sci; 5: 77-84. 1980.

training advice to go along with the charts.

Finally, a number of researchers (most notably Dr. Veronique Billat) have made the case that training at the velocity/power associated with your VO₂max (vVO₂max) is an excellent way of both raising VO₂max and the time you can spend at VO₂max. I agree with that notion. We will discuss the structures of workouts in that vein in the next chapter. Finding out your vVO₂max isn't quite as easy as reading it off a chart, but I think it is worth the trouble. See the fun activity boxes for more information. The original Montreal protocol was shown to be highly correlated with the "real" vVO₂max as measured with gas analysis gear.

> **Fun Activity #3:**
> Figure out your vVO₂max for swimming.
>
> 1. Bring a helper and a stopwatch to the pool.
> 2. Swim at your easiest pace.
> 3. Accelerate by 5-10 seconds/100M every 2 minutes. Have your helper signal you when you need to speed up. Your helper should record your 25 meter splits.
> 4. Your helper should signal you to stop when you are no longer maintaining pace. Your fastest sustained 2 minute speed is your vVO₂max.
>
> Adapted from: Leger and Boucher. An indirect running multistage field test, the Universite de Montreal Track Test. Can J Appl Sports Sci; 5: 77-84. 1980.

How do I figure out my LT without a lab test?

Unfortunately, you can't; at least not precisely. You will hear about something called the "Conconi Test" for figuring out LT. We will not discuss it because it has been shown to be a poor test. In other words, the only people who get any replicable results are people from Dr. Conconi's lab![4] You might as well just guess. It can occur anywhere between 70-90% of your maximal heart rate, with lower or higher values certainly possible. Another option would be to attempt to monitor you for the VT, or ventilatory threshold. Various coaches advocate ways to estimate this, but none are particularly accurate. In most people, the VT is associated with the lactate threshold, but this changes with training status.[5] Again, not a great marker; or rather, it is a reasonable marker in and of itself, but it is not an optimal marker for figuring out the LT. (Interestingly, it was initially thought that this phenomenon was due to the fact that lactate accumulation caused the blood to become more acidic, and that the body tried to compensate by exhaling something else acidic, CO_2. This is now known to be false, because people with McArdle's Disease, who are unable to make lactate, also have a ventilatory threshold).

As above, you really have only one viable alternative if you can't or don't want to do an invasive test: a functional test. You can perform an hour long time trial on your bike, or while running, or a 1500M swim. The idea is to perform the said task at the fastest pace you can maintain for the whole of the test. This will probably take you a few tries, as you will initially try to go out too hard and you will wear out too quickly. When you finally get this exercise down, you will have a good idea of your "threshold pace." This will correlate better with MLSS or OBLA, and will be higher than your pure "LT." However, it will get you into the ballpark.

Again, the benefit of this sort of field test is that it is functional, that is, it involves you on your bike (or running/swimming) the way you would in a race, without any labs or treadmills. It is more like the real thing. Also, these sorts of exercises help you learn to judge your own exertion. I have asked athletes in testing to tell me when they think they are near their threshold work load. More often than not, they are close. In fact, there was a paper by Stoudemire et al in 1996 showed that runners on a treadmill could adjust the treadmill speed to keep them at a pace close to their lactate threshold based on their subjective feelings.[6] The study subjects were only "recreationally active" as well, so it would seem you do not need a great deal of experience to be able to do this. However, please note that the subjects were "feeling" a blood lactate concentration between 2.5 mmol/L and 4 mmol/L. This seems in line with my experience, as tested athletes seem to associate "threshold" pace with a slightly greater effort level than that which elicits their initial bump in lactate.

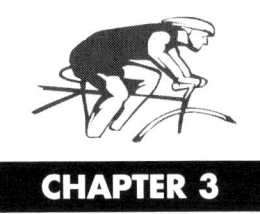

CHAPTER 3

What Kinds of Workouts Train Which Energy System?

It is important to make the point that exercise really falls on a continuum, and we can't divide it up without being sort of arbitrary. For example, doing workouts to increase your lactate threshold will also increase your VO2max, to some extent. On the other hand, a VO2max workout will by default also raise your lactate threshold somewhat. With that being said, let's get on to the nitty gritty of training and keep in mind that when we are talking about different workouts we are saying that the given protocol trains primarily the system in question, but also has some other effects as well.

Dr. Andrew Coggan wrote a chapter for US Cycling Expert Coaching Manual entitled *Training and Racing Using a Power Meter: An Introduction*, where he includes a couple of charts that indicate which physiologic parameters are most affected by what level of effort. Although it primarily deals with cycling, I highly recommend it. Dr. Coggan essentially defines 7 levels of intensity. I am going to go out on a limb and suggest that we only deal with those that affect our triathlon performance. (In other words, training for a 10 second, all out sprint at the end of a bike race is silly because it is unlikely we will ever use that skill in a triathlon, and we could use that training time to work on something that will be more valuable to us.) He defines the levels both in percentage of power at lactate threshold, and as a percentage of the heart rate at lactate threshold. I think this is particularly useful,

CHAPTER 3
What Kinds of Workouts Train Which Energy System?

Table 3.0 Exercise power and/or pace and corresponding expected physiologic adaptations.

Level 1	**Recovery**
%LTHR	<69%
%LT Pace	>125%
% vVO2max	>135%
%LT Power	<56%
Key Concept(s)	Promotion of circulation, glycogen restoration and repair; *rest without inactivity.*
Specific Adapt.	None

Level 2	**Endurance**
%LTHR	69-83%
%LT Pace	124-115%
%vVO2max	134-125%
%LT Power	56-75%
Key Concept(s)	Improvement of slow twitch fiber fatigue resistance; *Length more important than intensity.*
Specific Adapt.	Minimal improvement in oxidative enzyme levels
	Minimal improvement in LT
	Minimal Improvement in glycogen storage capacity
	Minimal conversion of Type IIb to Type IIa fibers

Level 3	**Tempo**
%LTHR	84-94%
%LT Pace	114-105%
%vVO2max	124-115%
%LT Power	76-90%
Key Concept(s)	Long race pace training: Marathon/IM/Half-IM. *Do not spend significant time here unless racing longer events.*
Specific Adapt.	Maximal improvement in glycogen storage capacity
	Moderate improvement in oxidative enzyme levels
	Moderate improvement in LT
	Moderate conversion of Type IIb to Type IIa fibers
	Minimal improvement in Type I hypertrophy
	Minimal improvement in muscle capillarization
	Minimal improvement in cardiac output
	Minimal improvement in VO2max
	Minimal improvement in plasma volume

CHAPTER 3
What Kinds of Workouts Train Which Energy System?

Level 4   **LT**
%LTHR   95-105%
%LT Pace   104-95%
%vVO2max   114-105%
%LT Power   91-105%
Key Concept(s)   Maximize metabolic fitness of muscles; *critical for all endurance race distances.*
Specific Adapt.   Maximal improvement in LT
                   Maximal improvement in oxidative enzyme levels
                   Moderate improvement in glycogen storage capacity
                   Moderate conversion of Type IIb to Type IIa fibers
                   Moderate improvement in cardiac output
                   Moderate improvement in VO2max
                   Moderate improvement in plasma volume
                   Minimal improvement in Type I hypertrophy
                   Minimal improvement in muscle capillarization

Level 5   **VO2max**
%LTHR   >106%
%LT Pace   94-84%
%vVO2max   104-95%
%LT Power   106-120% *or measured power at VO2max +/- 5%*
Key Concept(s)   Maximize cardiac fitness; *important for all endurance race distances.*
Specific Adapt.   Maximal improvement in VO2max
                   Maximal improvement in cardiac output
                   Maximal increased plasma volume
                   Moderate improvement in muscle capillarization
                   Moderate improvement in Type I hypertrophy
                   Minimal conversion of Type IIb to Type IIa fibers
                   Minimal improvement in oxidative enzyme levels
                   Minimal improvement in glycogen storage capacity

Data from: Daniels (1998), Coggan (2003), Billat (2000, 2003).

since the lactate threshold is the system we are most interested in optimizing for triathlon performance.

A. Training Your VO₂max

As you might guess, working at different levels of intensity will result in very different body adaptations. Fortunately, a lot off eggheads in a lot of labs have figured out what kinds of training improve each parameter. Let's talk about VO₂max to start out, since it is the most easily, or rather the most quickly, trained.

There is a particular method of training that you are going to quickly become familiar with, if you are not already. It is called interval training (figure 3.0). It was extensively described in the literature by a famous physiologist named Astrand, although there were certain people using it as a training technique much earlier. He illustrated that you do more work if you break it up. An example: take Eddie and Cletus. Let's put Eddie on a treadmill and let's tell him to go as hard as he can for a half hour. Let's put Cletus on the another treadmill and tell him to go just as hard for 30 seconds, but then run easy for 30 seconds, and repeat for a half hour or so. Then, let's order a couple pizzas to taunt them with and poke them with sharp sticks if we think they are slacking. Well, Eddie is going to get upset with us because he won't be able to go much longer than about ten or fifteen minutes. On the other hand, Cletus (with some poking) might well finish out the half hour. If we compare the amount of work both have done, we

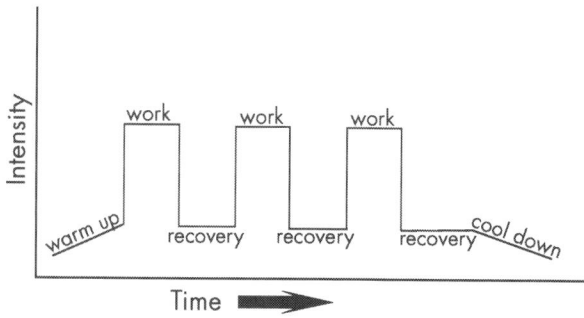

Figure 3.0   Schematic representation of interval training.

CHAPTER 3
What Kinds of Workouts Train Which Energy System?

will see that Cletus has done more total work than Eddie. What's more, Cletus will recover quicker than Eddie.

We can use interval workouts of different work and rest durations to improve many facets of your physiology, but right now we are talking about VO_2. Back in 1998, there was a study done in Japan which found that interval workouts consisting of 20 seconds of all out cycling, followed by 10 seconds of rest, for about 20 minutes a week improved VO_2max by 15%.[7] They also found that 60 minutes of easier exercise (they had the cyclists work at 70% of VO_2max) 5 times per week increased the VO_2 by almost 9%. There are two lessons to be learned here: you can increase your VO_2 with some minimal hard training, but your VO_2 will also improve appreciably (although not as much) with basic, uncomplicated training. My opinion is that you might as well spend 20 minutes a week and squeeze out the extra 6%.

> **VO_2 type intervals** work by increasing the pumping capacity of the heart.

The question you ought to be asking is, "Why does this work?" Earlier, we said that VO_2max is a function of how much blood the heart can deliver to working muscle. This is a simplification, but will do for our purposes. VO_2 type intervals work by increasing the pumping capacity of the heart through something called the Frank/Starling mechanism, which basically states that your heart responds to the stress you put on it. More specifically, it works like this: you start hammering away. Your muscles require more oxygen to get the increased work done, so they "tell" the local blood vessels (the capillaries) to open up by a special signaling mechanism. Your heart begins to pump harder and faster, to fill to dilating capillaries. Remember, your circulation is just that: a circuit. What gets pumped out must come back to the heart. The increase in blood return to the heart causes the walls of the heart to stretch. Frank/Starling states that the heart (when functioning properly) will eject what you put into it. And so on.

CHAPTER 3
What Kinds of Workouts Train Which Energy System?

Eventually, your heart improves itself by hypertrophy. In other words, it gets bigger and stronger, just like any muscle. This is why if you take an x-ray of a well trained endurance athlete, they often have a big heart. In fact, in the old days, there was some discussion in the medical field as to whether the "athletic heart" was some sort of disease process to be avoided. A second adaptation that occurs is plasma expansion. This simply means that your body increases the liquid portion of your blood (the plasma), which carries your red blood cells. This allows your heart to eject more blood with each beat.

Unfortunately, there are no studies I know of which show the specific optimal recipe for a VO_2 workout, so you will need to allow me a little latitude here. Above, we discussed how training improves your VO_2max. The truth is that it takes you a little while to ramp your heart rate and VO_2 up when increasing effort. For example, if you get up from the couch and sprint for the fridge, your heart rate response will lag your effort by a few seconds. It is probably safe to assume that work periods of 2-5 minutes at a heart rate within 10 beats or so of your max will be efficacious, with a minute or two of rest between. If you know about what workload your VO_2max occurs at, that is probably hard enough. The above period of time allows for your heart to come up to speed and start working hard, giving it the stimulus it needs to adapt.

The Japanese protocol probably sounds easier to you (20 sec work/10 sec rest). It obviously works as well, probably because you still ramp your heart rate / oxygen uptake up over time, and don't really give it much time to slow down with rest, so the net result is the same. Dr. Veronique Billat, a very well-respected exercise physiologist from France, is a proponent of the 30-30 protocol: 30 seconds of work, and 30 of recovery, repeated many times over.[8] (Note that Billat suggests the intervals be done at the lowest velocity which elicits VO_2max, rather than simply exercising at some difficult arbitrary velocity which is above it.) As I said above, there are no hard and fast rules here. Each of us is unique

CHAPTER 3
What Kinds of Workouts Train Which Energy System?

and we need to find what works for us. For novice athletes, I recommend the 30-30 (or similar) approach to VO$_2$max training, since it is relatively low impact and well tolerated. It is a good place to start, because it is less likely to get you hurt than running longer intervals, which can make you more tired, cause your form to break down, and allow you to make a mistake that injures you. It is also used by many much more experienced athletes.

Another benefit of the 30-30 protocol (or almost any protocol which has short work and rest durations) is that the athlete spends more time actually at VO$_2$max than they do with longer intervals. Billat has shown that spending more time at VO$_2$max, even if that total time is broken up over many small intervals, seems to increase the length of time an athlete is able to remain at VO$_2$max when the time comes for the athlete to do that for a longer period. The germane question is this: do we believe that total time spent at VO$_2$max is more important than the athlete doing the more "specific" training of fewer, more extended periods at VO$_2$max? I don't have a good answer to that question, because those experiments have not been done. For now, there are two schools of thought: the short repeat fans (Billat, Tabata and a few others) and those who favor the longer intervals (almost everyone else).

It is important to note that strengthening your heart does not mean that you will automatically reach your VO$_2$max. Cardiac output is the main determinant of VO$_2$max, but you need to train your muscles to be able to take maximal advantage of the work your heart is able to do. One way this happens is through an increase in the amount of capillaries, that is, the tiniest blood vessels that directly interact with the muscle fibers and drop off the oxygen they require. As your muscles develop more of these tiny blood vessels, your heart gets stronger and is able to fill them. The cycle continues until eventually your heart gets to the point that it cannot deliver any more blood. This is the point of VO$_2$max.

There is another portion to the VO$_2$ story, which we alluded to earlier: the "slow component" of VO$_2$. Recall that we stated that once an athlete crosses the lactate threshold, oxygen uptake begins to climb, even though work load is not. So as it turns out, it is possible not only to raise the maximal O_2 consumption, but to decrease this slow rise in oxygen consumption during exercise done below your maximum consumption. In a study by Carter and colleagues in 2000, it was shown that endurance run training combining 1-2 interval sessions/week above lactate threshold with running near lactate threshold 2-3 sessions/week could increase LT by 4% and VO2max by 3%.[9] No surprise there, other than these numbers were less than other studies had shown. (To be fair, the study subjects were already well trained and so we might not expect a large increase). What was interesting was that there was an average of a 35% decrease in the slow component of VO_2 at the same pace. In other words, they were using less oxygen to do the same amount of work and it took them longer to creep up to the level of their VO2max. So it would seem that working near your VO2max also makes you somewhat more efficient. We will get deeper into the idea of efficiency later.

> **Working near your VO2max** can also improve efficiency.

B. Training the Lactate Threshold

We have established the case that we can increase your VO2max in short period of time. That does not mean you get to hang up your shoes and call it at day after a few months. We still need to talk about training your lactate threshold, so that you can raise the amount of sustained work you can do. Consider this: if my VO2max is higher than yours, and our other characteristics are about the same, I should theoretically be able to do more work than you and beat you in a short race. However, suppose our race was several hours long, and suppose that my VO_2 was still higher than yours and I never worked on my lactate threshold, but you did. Like the proverbial tortoise and the hare, I would race off, and tire out quickly, whereas you could select a steadier, fast pace and blow by me after the first couple of miles while I was dragging my spaghetti legs down the road after you.

So, how do we train the lactate threshold? There was an excellent review of the subject written by Londeree in 1997, and it provided both good news and bad news.[10] Basically, Londeree analyzed more than 80 study groups statistically, looking at oxygen consumption and lactate concentration over several exercise intensity levels which ranged from sub-threshold to maximal. He also looked at the differences in the response to training between conditioned and sedentary subjects. What he found was that training at or near LT provided a good stimulus, and significantly increased the LT of sedentary subjects. The bad news was that such training resulted in insignificant gains in well conditioned study subjects. However, such subjects tended to respond better to higher levels of exercise. In other words, there is no free lunch, and this work confirmed that which was already probably intuitively clear to us. The better we get, the harder we must work to realize additional gains. (Interestingly, this correlates with what is known in the strength training literature: inexperienced weight lifters achieve the best gains by training with weights at 60% of their maximal lift ability, but better trained lifters see the best gains at 80% of their maximal lift ability).[11]

A study by Demarle and Colleagues in 2003 looked at several measures of athletic performance, including the VO2max, the speed at VO2max, the lactate threshold, the speed at LT, the economy of running, and the time to exhaustion in a maximal run test after an interval training program.[12] What they found was that all performance parameters were increased after 8 weeks of interval training in 7 subjects who had previously been sedentary. In the six well trained subjects, the improvements were less dramatic, with only about a 3% improvement in the speed of running at VO2max. This data correlates with the above study. Interestingly, in half of the well trained subjects (the three who improved their speed at LT), their time to

> **Increasing the velocity at LT is a major factor in improving performance.**

exhaustion during the maximal running test was improved by 10%, 24%, and 101%. The authors conclude that increasing the velocity at lactate threshold is a major factor in improving performance, especially in instances where you will be exercising at or above the lactate threshold.

So we have established that if we want to improve our lactate threshold as well as our performance, we need to train at or near our lactate threshold. It should also be clear that we need to spend a significant amount of time at or near lactate threshold. Exercise physiologist and elite cyclist Dr. Andrew Coggan advocates exercise bouts of 2x20 minutes at lactate threshold.[13] This is fine for cycling; however, I might consider shorter intervals for running and swimming as these activities can cause a little more wear and tear. I say this because running is quite high impact, and swimmers begin to lose form with fatigue and run the risk of straining something. Varying the actual length of the intervals within a few minutes of this is probably not going to make a huge difference. However, realize that the longer the exercise bout, the better you are training yourself for your races (presumably, if you are racing sprint triathlon you can expect to be spending most or all of your race near or above lactate threshold).

What are the end results of lactate threshold training? It will firstly reduce your body's production of lactate for a given workload.[14] It does this by causing your body to increase production of certain enzymes in your muscles, which allow a shift in your fuel balance to use more fat and less glycogen. Secondly, lactate threshold training will improve you body's ability to clear lactate.[15] Finally, it will increase the absolute amount of lactate you can tolerate before exhaustion, however, it should be noted that this change is minimal, and would be better realized through sprint-type training.[16] It should also be noted that such sprint-type training (i.e. what you would do to race the 100M dash) will do very little to improve your triathlon performance, since you spend very little time in triathlon in full out effort.

C. Training VO₂max When LT should be more important?

Again, it should be noted that while training at/near LT is probably the fastest/most efficient way of training LT, it is not the only means of doing so. Remember, exercise is a continuum and workouts below or above LT will still serve to improve the LT to some extent. As we recently discussed, the more experienced and better trained the athlete, the less they respond to training at LT. We also learned that the more trained athletes responded better to higher intensity exercise. Apparently, the top-level athletes have already discovered this. In a 2001 paper by Billat et al, the authors discuss the fact top class marathoners train in a very polarized fashion.[17] In other words, they do very little specific "LT" training, and instead train long distances at lower speeds, and do their faster training at speeds closer to what they would run for a 1.5k or 10k race. They still do a little LT work, but only perhaps once per week and only at the tail end of a longer distance workout.

Billat has several possible explanations for this. Chiefly, she hypothesizes that this type of schedule reduces the risk of overtraining, which seems to be more of a risk when daily training becomes too monotonic at too high an intensity. In other words, miles and miles at or above lactate threshold may simply wear the athlete out. I believe there is some sense to this, not only physiologically but also psychologically. Again, it will be up to the athlete and coach to decide what stimulus serves to improve performance best. Interestingly, Paula Radcliffe has, in recent years, been a dominant force in running over middle distance (i.e. 10k) and long distance (the marathon). It would seem that therefore that success in middle and long distance does not necessarily need to be mutually exclusive; even if marathon speed ought to be close to LT velocity and 10k speed ought to be closer to velocity at VO₂max (table 3.1).

Table 3.1 Paula Radcliffe's 2002 race times

Date	Race	Distance	Place	Time
March 23	Cross Country Worlds	8k	1st	26:55
April 14	London Marathon	42k	1st	2:18:56
July 28	Commonwealth Games	5k	1st	14:31
Aug. 6	European Championship	10k	1st	30:01
Oct. 12	Chicago Marathon	42k	1st (WR)	2:17:18

There is an argument to be made for the idea that training at the velocity associated with VO2max is important for highly trained athletes.[19] The theory is that peripheral, rather than central factors are limiting performance in such athletes. For example, Dr. Billat hypothesizes that interval training at vVO2max improves the aerobic potential of the Type IIA (fast twitch, oxidative) fibers, making them more fatigue resistant.[20] There is some sense to this thought.

I tell you this in the interest of completeness, however, I think it would be reckless to abandon/severely limit LT work in favor of VO2max work when training for triathlon, especially over the longer (half-IM to IM) distances, and especially since most of us are not competing at the level of the so-called top class marathoner. I would, however, consider including a greater proportion of these types of workouts (30-30) in the instance of the extremely well trained (elite or high level age-group) athlete who seemed to have reached a plateau on a steady diet of distance work and solid lactate threshold training over a period of years.

D. Training Endurance Capacity

Earlier we said that you would need to do some specific endurance type workouts, because you cannot keep doing LT and VO2max intervals constantly and keep functioning. (Well, that might be a bit of an overstatement. If the athlete was extremely well trained, and careful to remain just at or immediately below LT, and did little VO2max work, it is likely they could proceed in that way for quite some time.) That being said, remember the

CHAPTER 3
What Kinds of Workouts Train Which Energy System?

longer / slower workouts we term "endurance workouts" will in fact serve to help raise your LT and even VO_2 to some extent, but by now you understand that this would not be the most efficient ways of training those parameters.

So what are we talking about when we speak about training for "endurance?" Here, we are focusing more on the concept of distance than on a high pace. Most physiology texts indicate that you achieve much of the physiologic gain of a particular training volume or intensity after 4-6 weeks of training at that level. To achieve further adaptation, either pace must be improved or volume must be increased. In my experience as a physician, there comes a point when additional intensity is riskier than it is worth. In other words, the intensity is near the fine balance point of training vs. injury. That extra interval may give you the extra few seconds in a race, and it may also pull a hamstring that will result in impressive detraining while you are recovering.

The most impressive volumes of training are often done by professional cyclists, who may ride more than 35,000 kilometers (about 25,500 miles) per year.[21] It has also been shown that these athletes are often able to work at very high workloads for long periods of time, without any apparent fatigue of the slow twitch muscle units.[22] Also, professional road cyclists have a less impressive rise in their slow component of VO_2, around 7.6 ml/min, when compared to untrained people, around 22 ml/min.[23] In my mind, this indicates a couple of things. Firstly, the principle of specificity (that the body adapts precisely to the stimulus provided) suggests that long miles at a lower intensity will serve to more exclusively train the slow twitch motor units. Since

> **Don't overlook** your slow miles because you'd rather do more exciting interval training.

the slow component is generally attributed to the recruitment of fast twitch fibers as the slow twitch fibers get tired, we can by inference consider that this extremely small slow component is secondary to very strong and fatigue resistant slow fibers. In other words, don't overlook your slow miles because you'd rather do more exciting interval training. There is likely significant value to the "endurance workout."

E. Training Efficiency and Economy

This will be a very short section. You have been blessed with a brain and a system of nerves that constantly talks to it. In a manner of speaking, you are constantly self-coaching. What I mean by this is the following: if you look at well trained runners, what you find is that most of them automatically select the most economical cadence and stride length for their body type and fitness.[24]

This makes good sense if you think about it. Back in prehistoric times, when our mammalian ancestors needed to worry about things like running away from saber toothed tigers and whatnot; it helped to be as quick as possible. There were no long-haired scientists and physicians loafing around stroking their goatees and hypothesizing ways to make people faster. People weren't out at the track running intervals. So, slow people got eaten and fast people survived long enough to have babies, and the faster of those babies survived, and so on. The brain developed a means of self correcting your mechanics to make the best of what you had. What I am saying is that there probably is not a whole lot of sense trying to alter the way you run if you have been doing it for any length of time, at least in physiologic terms. In medical terms, however, a physician specialist might watch you run and make suggestions based on your pain or injury patterns. The best advice across the board is probably "If it isn't broken, don't fix it."

Increase in running speed is largely due to an increase in stride length. However, it is important to realize that this generally results in a higher oxygen uptake for a given pace, and thus reduced economy.[25] Now, you could argue that we are not interested in having the most economical performance; we are interested in maximizing our performance regardless of cost because our goal is to get to the finish line as quickly as possible. There is some sense to this line of thinking. However, remember that a key feature in the ability to win many running races (and cycling races, for that matter) is the ability to lift the pace in the final stages of the race[26], which you might not be able to do if you are too fatigued from earlier difficult efforts.

The relevant question is this: will your performance benefit from remaining economical for the greater portion of the race, minimizing energy expenditure, and making a move at the end, or from racing from the front? This depends on several factors: for example, the format of the race. In a time trial format, your goal is to get to the finish at your personal fastest possible pace, and hope this happens to be faster than everyone else. (This presupposes that you are not the last rider to go, in which case you would know just how fast you needed to go and could judge accordingly.) In a pure group race format, your goal is to get to the finish line first. Whether or not you achieve your personal maximal performance is not necessarily relevant unless you are attempting to break some sort of record.

You must also consider your particular physiology and training status. For example, Paula Radcliffe set the world record at the 2002 Chicago Marathon by running from the front. I suspect that if tested, we would have found that she had a higher lactate threshold than her competition, was working at a relatively lower percentage of her VO$_2$max at her given pace, and was thus more economical and able to dominate from the beginning. (She was, in fact, also able to lift her pace in the final miles, however, this was not instrumental to her win as she was already far out in front.) Contrast this strategy with her performance in the 2000 Olympic 10k, where she attempted to run from the front at what might have been too high a pace, and found that she was unable to match the moves of her competitors in the final moments. We cannot know if she was in her optimal training state, or if there were other physical or psychological factors involved, of course. Assuming that her increased speed was due to longer/less economic stride length, might she have benefited from sitting in the pack, remaining closer to her most economical running parameters and watching her competition? Perhaps, though I suspect we should not do too much Monday morning quarterbacking; we can not know what she was feeling as the race unfolded. My point here is that you do not want to write a strategic check that your physiology cannot cash.

A point worth mentioning is that the gait cycle does not necessarily operate on the sole basis of optimizing economy. Dr. Billat has hypothesized that at higher speeds, the gait changes to lessen peak forces on the joints, serving as protection against injury at the expense of pure "economy." She bases this opinion on her own work and on some gait analysis of horses, where this phenomenon was first described. Again, we can take the long view that this improves economy overall, because it lessens the likelihood of injury and thus averts the very uneconomic activity of limping along through recovery. Thus, there may be some value to the sorts of drills and visualization running coaches tend to espouse, such as the "light footfall," or "running on eggshells." Though there is no data on whether these rather nebulous concepts can be taught, it is clear that athletes can be taught to alter their gait pattern. Whether this is a valuable enterprise, rather that simply allowing the body to do what it does, is anyone's guess. In the face of recurrent injury, it might be worth a try.

There is some discussion today regarding training the economy of cyclists. For example, many coaches advocate one legged cycling drills and the like. The general idea is that if the rider is able to "pedal circles," and use more muscles, rather than simply pushing on the down stroke and allowing the other leg to come up, he/she will be more efficient. However, there is precious little information to support efforts to actively train efficiency. A paper by Coyle and colleagues examined the biomechanical factors associated with elite cycling performance.[27] They compared the mechanics of national class cyclists with state class cyclists who were a little slower and found something very interesting. The cyclists of national caliber (who had generally been riding longer) generated more power than the other group. No surprise there.

However, they did it by applying more power on the down stroke, not by actively trying to "pedal circles" or "lift their feet" or unweight their pedals on the upstroke. This was surprising, since everyone always assumed that speed came from applying more force around the whole of the pedal stroke. It would seem that speed comes from practice through more years of riding, not necessarily trying to be more efficient through "drills."

This doesn't make a whole lot of sense to us, at least to those of us who have been training for years using the older philosophies of coaching. Many cycling books (and a number of coaches) suggest one legged drills, and there are even aftermarket cranks available that force you to pedal circles by disconnecting the pedals from one another. We need to think about the subject more deeply, considering the anatomy of our bodies and what "efficiency" really means.

There are a lot of muscles in your lower limbs, but we will discuss two groups: the knee extensors and the hip flexors. Your knee extensors are your quads. They are big, strong, and have been developed by Mother Nature for walking and running. They very efficiently straighten your leg. Your hip flexors, on the other hand, are very small muscles that serve to pick your leg up a few centimeters when you have to swing it forward when it is time to take the next step. On your bike, your quads are in a prime position to do a lot of work, in terms of their strength and optimal range of motion. Your hip flexors are in a very bad position in terms of their optimal strength and range of motion. Even when you are riding about as hard as you can, you aren't using all possible available power from your quads. So the question becomes, which is more "efficient" for your brain to do: use a little muscle and try to "round" your pedal stroke, or better use your big muscles that are able to generate many times the power.

Another point worth mentioning involves cadence, that is, the speed at which you are spinning your legs. Ever since Lance Armstrong started winning the Tour de France, much has been made by cycling commentators and coaches alike as to the benefits of "spinning;" that is, using a higher cadence than one might typically select. In 1998, Zoldadz and colleagues did experiments analyzing cadence, lactate, oxygen uptake and efficiency while keeping power output (the actual amount of work done) constant.[28] What they found was interesting. At 40, 60, 80 and 100 rpm, the above parameters remained fairly constant and well within the margin of measurement error. At 120 rpm, there was a large increase in the physiologic markers and a decrease in efficiency. In other words, they weren't doing any more work in terms of moving forward, but they were expending more energy, using more oxygen, and generating more lactate. Coupled with earlier research that shows that most people self-select their best cadence with training, this makes a good case for the notion that we should not be overzealous about training at higher and higher cadences.

Even Lance Armstrong has gone overboard with spinning. In a time trial at the 2002 Tour De France, his cadence, based on the video and his own account of the event indicate he was spinning between 110 and 120 rpm. He did not win the event, and afterwards, he stated that he thought he got "a little carried away" with his cadence. In the following time trial, it was reported that he had a cadence sensor placed on the bike to make sure he stayed in a reasonable range. This is not particularly scientific, but it might make us a little suspicious based on what we now know about cadence.

Unfortunately, we cannot use the same rules for swimming. Your brain developed primarily for two legged movements on dry land. The bicycle just happens to take advantage of the way your body is built and your brain is wired. Swimming, on the other hand, is a very unnatural motion. Thus, if you want to become a better swimmer, you are most likely going to need to invest in lessons from a good coach who can give you feedback on your form. Once you develop good mechanics, your brain will take over and the motions will become natural, and you will get better and better through practice doing precisely what you ought to do: swimming. A lot. Why, you may ask? We will cover that in the next chapter.

I've stopped getting faster! How do I alter my program?

This is a question I often get from people who are self coaching, and it does in fact fall squarely in the realm of coaching. It cannot be answered without a detailed analysis of the athlete, and his/her training program, diet and goals. Most people asking this question feel they are "plateauing," that is, they are not seeing improvement even though they continue to train. There are several possibilities here. The first is that they have reached their genetic limitations. I suspect this is the vast minority of cases, and I have not yet had the privilege of meeting at athlete at that level. The second is that the athlete has reached the limit of what they can accomplish with the time he or she has available. This is more common. The third is that the athlete needs a significant change in stimulus. This is most common, in my experience.

It is of paramount importance that a change be made logically. Let's consider a triathlete who feels she or she is not improving: firstly, we want to look for the limiter. In other words, is the athlete significantly behind the curve in one area? If so, we might consider adding a workout in that particular sport, while putting the other two into maintenance phase. For example, the athlete might be a career swimmer and long time runner who is able to run/swim in the top 25th percentile, but is a less accomplished cyclist, perhaps the 50th percentile. We could add an additional cycling workout and likely subtract 1 or two other workouts without great detriment.

What if the athlete feels that he/she is tiring prematurely after move to longer distances in racing? We might wonder if the athlete overzealous, exercising too hard and running down his/her glycogen stores early on. (For the moment, let us imagine the athlete is consuming a proper diet.) We might be tempted to increase training distance, or increase the LT workouts. However, we must be cautious not to simply pile on easy mileage. Remember, we want our training to be directed, that is, we should always be mindful that we have a specific goal in mind. Astrand has stated that exercise must elicit at least 50% of VO2max, and preferably 70-80% as the athlete progresses, to see any increase in fitness.[29] Assuming the athlete has more time to train, and is currently subscribing to a well balanced plan, we might consider sensibly-applied additional volume at LT effort during long training days, but decrease the total distance covered. Why? These workouts serve to improve metabolic fitness. As fitness improves the athlete will now be exercising at a lower metabolic cost for the same speed. Thus, he or she should spare more glycogen, burn more fat, and increase time to fatigue. Would this work? It might, or might not. I have seen both results. However, the germane point is that we are making a specific intervention to correct the problem we perceive, rather than simply throwing miles at the problem and leaving the athlete's body to sort it out. Further, if it does not work, we know the one thing we changed, and can now change another parameter and monitor for the response we desire.

Above all, if through careful analysis one determined a need for more intensity, I would then advocate for small stepwise increases in the length of time spent on intense (VO2max) workouts, depending upon what the athlete was able to tolerate. I would be very cautious about arbitrarily attempting to train at a faster pace. This is generally the pattern I see in athletes who have become injured, or who are about to. That being said, there is evidence showing that people not responding to one particular regimen can benefit from a change. In a study of cross country skiers, Gaskill et al showed that athletes who did not respond to a program of high volume, low intensity workouts were able to increase their performance by changing the percentages of train-

> **Be very cautious** about arbitrarily attempting to train at a faster pace.

ing.[30] By raising their level of high intensity training from 17% of total training time to 35%, they were able to increase their VO2max by 9% and their arm power by 18%.

Again, I am not suggesting an arbitrary jump to more intense training if your current program is not working. To paraphrase a noted exercise physiologist and running coach Dr. Jack Daniels, don't leave your race on the training track. Training is best done patiently; we are not looking for maximal immediate goals, but for steady sustainable improvement a bit at a time. Your physiology cannot continually make the quantum leaps in performance that you made when you first started training. You are setting yourself up for failure if you try. It is better for you to spend the requisite time in trial and error "paying your dues" until you find your optimal regimen than for you to spend time injured and wondering how you could have prevented it.

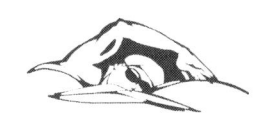

CHAPTER 4

The Underlying Principle of Training: Specificity

With regards to your training, the most important concept I can convey to you is that of specificity, which we began touching on in the last chapter. What this means is that your body will adapt precisely to the stress you put upon it. In other words, if you want to get good at basketball, you have to shoot a lot of hoops. Riding your bike isn't going to make you a better power forward.

There has been much research on the subject of specificity. A classic paper was written by Magel and colleagues in January of 1975.[31] They had fifteen college age swimmers (recreational swimmers, not swim team members) begin swimming intervals for 1 hour per day, 3 days per week, for 10 weeks. They checked VO₂max both in the water and on a running treadmill before and

> **Your body will adapt precisely to the stress you put upon it.**

after they did the training program. What they found was that the swimming program significantly increased VO₂max while swimming by 380 ml/minute. However, their VO₂max measured when running showed no change. This experiment showed that the training for a sport was specific to that sport, and would not necessarily transfer to other sports.

It is easy to see the difference in that example, because swimming and running are very different activities. But what about the difference between, say, running and cycling?

We might reason that running and cycling use many of the same muscles, so perhaps we can train on the bike and become better runners. This seems reasonable on the surface. In fact, for an untrained person, there is some truth to this statement. Earlier we talked about how the body adapts to exercise through changes in the cardiovascular system. If you were a couch potato, and we put you on a bike for an hour a day a few times per week, and stuck you with something pointy if you tried to slow down, you would have some solid workout time. If after a month of this, we took you out to a track and made you run a mile, we would almost certainly find that you were now able to run faster than you could before we made you train on the bike. The key in this example is that we started with an untrained person, for whom *any* training stimulus (even weight lifting) will enhance cardiac performance enough that we could detect the improvement in other areas.

A good study for comparison was done by Coyle and colleagues in 1991.[32] What these guys did was take a group of well trained cyclists who were about the same age. They separated the cyclists into groups who had been training for about ten years, and those who had been training for about five. They measured the VO_2max of these people on the bike, and found that in general the more experienced riders had higher VO_2's, and were better trained. This stands to reason: they have been training longer, so they *should* be fitter. Now, what happens if you put them on a treadmill and measure their VO_2? It turns out that both groups were all pretty quick, but they *all* had the *same* VO_2 when running as hard as they could. So we discovered something important. No matter how much bike training you do, even 5 years extra, it isn't going to make you a better runner. (Again, assuming you are not a couch potato).

Another good example of specificity has been exhibited in one-legged training experiments done by Costill.[33] Basically, if you exercise one leg on a bike and leave the other alone, you notice something interesting. When you test lactate threshold and VO_2 using the trained leg, you find that both parameters have improved. If you test the non-trained leg, you find no improvement in VO₂ or LT, even though you have been training the cardiac system through exercise. Why is this? It is true that training has the central effect of improving how much blood your heart can pump, no matter what you are exercising. However, recall that we earlier stated that there are specific changes in the muscles you exercise. Your muscle cells generate enzymes in response to exercise which help transport and dispose of lactate. They shift their metabolism to rely more on fat at the same intensity, as we talked about earlier. Finally, your muscles build a larger network of capillaries that your heart can fill with blood to provide more oxygen. This is they key point: *to really achieve VO₂max, you need a strong heart coupled with strong muscles which you have specifically trained to work with it.* Ergo, maximal exercise capacity is absolutely linked to the specificity of training.

It is important to remember that specificity isn't just about local muscle changes. Remember, your brain is the conductor of your athletic train. It is the brain that determines the patterns and orders in which your muscles need to be firing to get you moving as quickly as possible. These patterns become ingrained and strengthened with training. They are corrected over time to maximize efficiency. Again, to use the example of running versus cycling, you are not necessarily recruiting your muscles in precisely the same way, even though you are using many of the same muscles. Also, you are using other muscles in different ranges of motion.

This neurological point can be nicely exemplified in weight lifting: there are great changes in strength in the short term (a few weeks), before there have been any significant modifications to the muscles themselves. How can this be? The athlete may not look different, but we cannot deny that their performance has increased tens of percentage points. This is due to better recruitment of the already-existing muscles and more organized firing patterns of the brain and nerves. Thus, it isn't just about exercising. It is about doing precisely the activity you are trying to improve so that you maximally train your brain, as well as your muscles.

CHAPTER 5

Strength Training

The short answer to the question, "Will strength training make me faster?" is probably no. The slightly longer answer is yes, if you are currently a couch potato. The longer answer is yes, if it keeps you from getting hurt. Surprisingly, there have not been many studies done to address the specific point that many coaches espouse: that weight training increases performance in endurance events. I will cover a few related papers, and suggest a review article for further study if you are interested.

By and large, studies that show an endurance performance benefit to weight training were carried out in untrained populations. For example, a 1991 paper by Marcinik and coworkers concluded that after a 12 week strength training program, previously untrained participants had a roughly 33% increase in time to fatigue while cycling at 75% of their VO_2max.[34] This group also had an increase in their LT of 12%. There was not an increase in VO_2max overall, however. Another study by McCartney et al in 1991 showed that patients with heart disease who trained for 10 weeks aerobically increased their cycling time at 80% of their maximal possible power by 11% (which was insignificant).[35] However, they also demonstrated that patients who added weight training to the regimen increased their maximal power by 109%. Again, the patients were untrained, and moreover, none of the participants went longer than approximately 10-12 minutes.

There are, in fact, a few studies which would seem to support weight training for endurance performance in people with at least some training under their belt. Some of the more relevant studies were carried out by Hickson and colleagues in 1988.[36] They evaluated 10 weeks of heavy resistance training in subjects who were already trained cyclists or runners. They found that while leg strength increased by an average of 30%, the oxidative enzyme (citrate synthase) activity they measured was not increased. Furthermore, cycling and running VO$_2$max values were unchanged. Cycling at 80% of VO$_2$max until exhaustion increased from 71 minutes to 85 minutes, while there was not any significant difference in 10k running times.

Bastiaans et al looked at replacing some endurance training with "explosive" weight training in trained cyclists in 2001.[37] His results were not impressive in terms of performance benefit, but that it was possible to replace 37% of a cyclists program with strength training and not negatively affect his/her endurance performance. This would seem to debunk the theory of an interference effect. This theory states that you can't do both weight training and endurance training at the same time if you want to do either properly, because one type interferes with the body adapting to the other. However, it should be noted that weight training to the point that you feel tired will have a negative impact on performance, because you will not be able to give 100% to your endurance workouts.

Swimmers often include weight training in their programs. Tanaka et al looked at competitive swimmers, who were matched for stroke and performance.[38] All swimmers participated in a similar swim program, while half of them added three sessions of weight training per week for 14 weeks, utilizing the major muscle groups used in the front crawl. The swimmers who trained with weights increased their strength by 25-35%; however, their swim performance was not improved.

Finally, there was an excellent review article on weight training and endurance performance written by John Hawley a couple of years ago. I highly recommend it to those of you curious enough to seek it out. He proposes several reasons for the observation that weights seem to help the untrained more than the trained.[39] First, these people will benefit from *any* stimulus which overloads the working muscles, since they are doing little to no exercise otherwise. Secondly, and more importantly, athletes with little training typically have poor technique; thus, they compensate through the application of more force. Well trained athletes can usually already generate large amounts of power, and thus their further improvements will come through refinement of technique. Hawley's paper concludes with his comment that "modern training studies do not support the use of resistance training programs for improving the performances of highly trained athletes." I must agree.

Now you are thinking, "Excellent! No more gym workouts!" Wrong. What I wrote was that weight training probably won't do much to improve your performance directly, unless you are what the researchers call an "untrained person." As a physician, I must still recommend some basic strength work. My job isn't necessarily to shave every last second off of your 10k time, but to keep you training consistently and more importantly, out of the doctor's office!

First and foremost, your joints are built to function optimally in a certain way; particular alignments of bones and joint articular surfaces function well in specific angles and ranges of motion. Muscular and tendinous strength and resilience are what put and keep them in the appropriate orientation. Earlier, we said that specific training strengthens the above structures such that they work best for that particular activity. But what happens when the unforeseen takes place and those structures are placed under unnatural forces?

Say you are trail running, lose your footing, and take a tumble. Perhaps you have to catch yourself by grabbing a branch. Whether or not you stop your fall before a season ending injury takes place will depend very little on your specific running strength and flexibility, and very much on your overall strength

CHAPTER 5
Strength Training

and agility. If your shoulder girdle muscles are strong enough to handle the sudden application of stress as you catch yourself, you may not be injured at all, or might perhaps suffer a minor strain. If they aren't, you might tear a muscle or tendon and be looking at surgery or extended rehab, not to mention the fact that you might have broken a bone, since you were unable to stop your fall. How much sport specific training will you be doing when you are casted and slung?

I am not suggesting that you go out and start lifting like a weight junkie. This would be absolutely counterproductive. What I am suggesting is that you have a basic, overall plan of strength and flexibility maintenance that does not detract too much from your primary goal of training from your specific sport. In your off season, maybe do a bit more strength work to break up the monotony of training you were involved in during the regular season. Lifting weights and doing strength exercises increases strength, but also increase flexibility. A study on rabbits which was presented some years ago demonstrated that stretching alone merely increased the length of stretch before failure of a tendon. However, studies using strength training throughout the range of motion increased length before failure *and* the amount of stress required to cause said failure.

> **I respectfully suggest to you that an uninjured athlete is faster than an injured one, and that moderate overall strength training with a decrease in intensity during the racing season might be just insurance you need.**

The bottom line is this: strength training will likely do little or nothing to improve your specific athletic performance directly. However, I respectfully suggest to you that an uninjured athlete is faster than an injured one, and that moderate overall strength training with a decrease in intensity during the racing season might be just the insurance you need.

CHAPTER 6

Detraining: What Happens When We Get Hurt, or Lazy

Astrand provides a nice discussion of the classic study which analyzed the effects of de- and re-training on relatively untrained subjects[40]. What I mean by that is that this study analyzed a few average people by making them train for 50 days, putting them on bed rest for 20 days, and then starting them training again. Five of these people were couch potatoes, and three of them were somewhat active.

Over the period of bed rest, all subjects lost approximately 27% of their maximal oxygen uptake. The amount of blood their heart was able to pump per beat also dropped about 25%. The heart rate required to achieve the same level of oxygen uptake went from 145 bpm to 180 bpm. In other words, this was a major loss of fitness. When the couch potato subjects began exercising again, they were able to achieve their trained level of function within 10 days, and after another 50 days of training had improved their VO$_2$max to a level higher than that seen at the end of their first 50 day training session.

The three previously trained subjects, who initially had much higher VO$_2$ values, never reduced their fitness to the level of the couch potato group; however, it took them 30 to 40 days to get back to the level they were at before the bed rest. This makes an important point. In absolute terms, the well trained athlete does not seem to come down to the level of the sedentary person after a period of deconditioning. However, it takes far longer for them

CHAPTER 6
Detraining: What Happens When We Get Hurt, or Lazy

to return to their previous level of fitness.

Earlier, we discussed the idea that there are two major enzymatic systems we are training, the ones that break down carbohydrate (glycolytic) and the ones that break down fats (oxidative). In 1984, Coyle et al analyzed the time course of the loss of adaptations in the oxidative systems. What he found was that two of the main oxidative enzymes he used as makers (citrate sythetase and succinate dehydrogenase) decreased over a period of a month and stabilized at a level 50% above that of sedentary individuals.[41] Interestingly, muscle capillarization did not decrease much with time, and remained 50% higher than that in sedentary individuals. Thus, it would seem that the ability of the muscles to do work decreases more dramatically than the infrastructure the body built to support them.

There are also central changes that take place with detraining. A review written by Mujika and Padilla in 2000 looked at the differences in detraining with short-term removal of exercise versus long term[42]. Again, within roughly four weeks there is a decrease in VO$_2$max. This is ascribed to a decrease in plasma (the liquid part of your blood that carries the red and white cells) volume. The problem is that your heart pumps less blood with each beat, and it cannot speed up enough to make up for this loss. Coyle, Hemmert and Coggan measured this decrease at roughly 12%.[43] They also found that there was a decrease in stroke volume of the heart by about 12%. Interestingly, they also found that you could reverse this change by infusing an equivalent amount of a saline/dextran solution. In fact, it was possible to return VO$_2$max to within 2-4% of trained values by this mechanism. Thus, we can surmise that part of the problem is that the body stops maintaining an excess of fluid to bolster the output of the heart when it is no longer necessary.

The take home message is that most of these changes are less pronounced the longer you have been training before you become detrained, with the exception of the decreases in plasma and thus stroke volume. However, those changes are the most quickly reversed. The athlete would do well to remember Astrand's admonition, however, which is that with age the athlete becomes harder and harder to train/re-train.[44] For example, athletes that never become detrained are often very successful racing at the highest levels of their sports into their late 30's. Vlatchislav Ekimov, a cyclist with US Postal, won the Olympic gold medal in the time trial at age 34, and returned to the Olympics to defend it at age 38, claiming the silver medal. Cyclists and other athletes who allow themselves to become detrained after retirement, and then make a "comeback" months or years later sometimes have a much harder time, if they are able to return at all. The good news is that it takes less work to maintain fitness for a period of time than it does to build (or re-build) it in the first place.

CHAPTER 7

Periodization: The Reductionist Viewpoint

Periodization is an important concept. The general idea is that you must make specific decisions regarding what kinds of training you will be doing at each point of the season, each building upon the one before. It is essential to realize that you can't arbitrarily throw together a bunch of workouts and perform optimally on race day. Inger has reported that cross-country skiers who did not periodize their training never reached the top levels of competition.[45] In fact, varying VO2max with the lowest values pre-competition and the highest values during the competitive season was very important to success.

With careful planning, you can ensure that your fitness improves steadily and that you come into competition at your peak, with a few caveats. There is not a vast body of literature researching the questions of optimal periodization for endurance athletes; only that it seems to be necessary for optimal performance. I suspect that this is because everyone's response to exercise is very different, and everyone has a different athletic history.

One thing most coaches and physiologists (including people who are both) would advise is that you should take the long view of training.[46, 47] If you make exercise a major part of your life over a period of years (which I recommend in terms of your health, as well as the enjoyment of sport), then you have the advantage of setting a long term goal for yourself. You also have the advantage of planning a steady climb towards your goal. An example of this

CHAPTER 7
Periodization: The Reductionist Viewpoint

is the runner looking forward to the next Olympics. To be sure, your long term goal need not be anything like the Olympics, but maybe you are at the beginning of your triathlon career and see an Ironman in your future. Take it from me: if you take a crack at something like Ironman without a long term plan, you may finish because you can gut it out. You may also prematurely end your athletic career, as I very nearly did some years ago.

The first thing to understand is that there is something called a "dose-response" relationship between training and performance (figure 7.0). It is actually a little bit more complicated than that, but this will suffice for the beginning explanation.[48] The training "dose" is equal to the intensity times the duration.[49] If you look at the graph, there is an amount of training that will provide you with the greatest "bang for your buck." A little more training will continue your improvements, but at a lesser rate. This is your

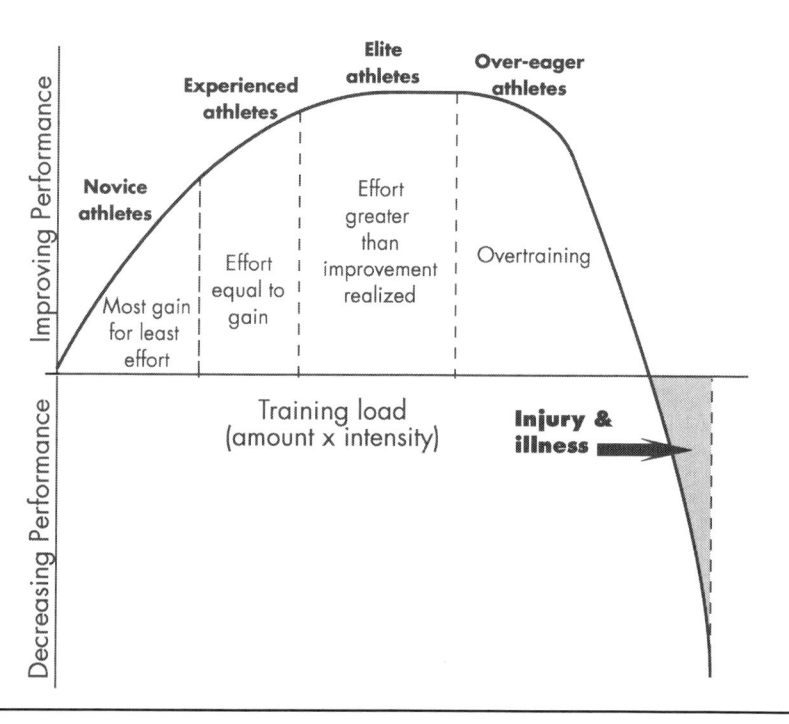

Figure 7.0 The relationship between training and performance. Adapted from: Noakes 2001, Busso 2003, and Morton 1990.

optimal training area. The next realm is that of diminishing returns; once you enter this area, you are beginning to risk running yourself down, rather than improving your form further. Finally, you enter an area where your athletic drive has outstripped your body's reserves of strength and durability.

Early in your career, it is my observation (and experience) that these zones are compressed. In other words, you will get the biggest returns on the smallest investment on just a few hours of training a week, you'll see the optimum benefits with an hour or two more, and you will begin to run your body down with any more. It will not always be this way. As you train more, the stronger you will get, and the more you will be able to train. The trick is to allow your body to keep up, and to advance on its terms, not the terms your brain would like it to.

Now, let us consider how we break the season up into periods or cycles. We can call the whole of the season the "macrocycle" (figure 7.1). This is made up of smaller periods, or "mesocycles." Earlier, we mentioned that full adaptation to a stimulus takes between 4 to 6 weeks, but can take as long as 8. Then, the stimulus must be altered if continued improvement is to be had. This provides the physiologic rationale dictating that we need to divide our long term plan into smaller chunks, and thus we can safely decide that our mesocycles can be 6 to 8 weeks in length. This

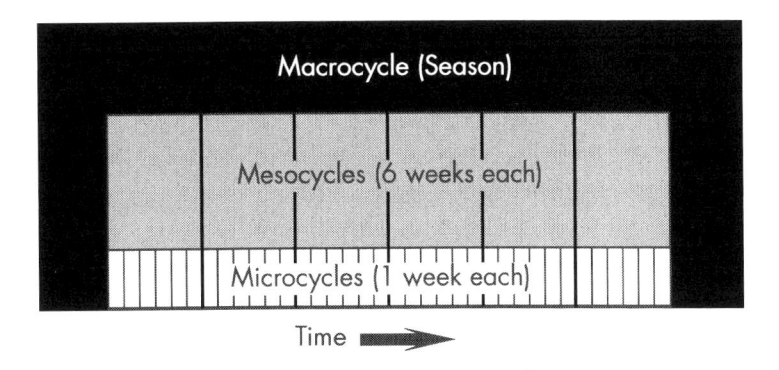

Figure 7.1   The relationship of the macrocycle to mesocycles and microcycles.

was nicely illustrated in a recent paper by Busso in 2003[48], who carried out a reasonably simple experiment. He found out the maximal power a cyclist could hold for 5 minutes, and then had them do a set of intervals at 85% of that power for 4 minutes, followed by three minutes of recovery. This was repeated several times over, and the workout was done 3 times a week. A couple times a week, the athletes did another test to find out the maximal power they could hold for 5 minutes, and this number was then used in the next training session. The athletes began to plateau between six and eight weeks, at an average of 27% improvement. At this point, the training sessions were increased to 5 times a week, which yielded an additional 3% improvement. These data also illustrate the point of crossover from the optimal training zone to that of diminishing returns.

We can now move into the smallest cycle, or microcycle; that is, the weekly schedule. It makes sense that we would not be doing ourselves any favors by stacking all of our difficult training in the space of a couple of days, because we would spend the rest of the week just trying to recover from them. The aforementioned Busso study (among others) developed complex equations to describe what is already intuitively obvious to anyone who has tried two hard workouts in a row: your response to each training "dose" is dependant upon the fatigue you are feeling from previous recent doses.[48,50] There must be a place for adequate recovery.

The confounding effect of fatigue is an important observation to make from Busso study.[50,51] That is, the athletes were training more, which should make them better, but when they were training more, they were overall more tired and were seeing diminished returns. What we seek to do is end each cycle before this point. At the time we begin to see the diminishing returns, we change the stimulus; not by simply adding more of the same, but putting the adaptations made in that period in "maintenance mode," and moving onto the next adaptation we seek.

Earlier, we laid out the course of changes in terms of amount of improvement, and the time scale of those improvements, for

CHAPTER 7
Periodization: The Reductionist Viewpoint

each energy system. It logically follows that we can use that information to our advantage in terms of deciding which order to put our various periods in. It is this reductionist mindset which keeps us from training aimlessly: we keep our long view in the back of our minds, but set up a series of periods as stepping stones to the long term goal.

For example, a hypothetical 5-10k runner might be interested in racing a half marathon, but might not be in the condition required to train for that distance. Thus, we make the half-marathon the focus of the macrocycle. In setting up the mesocycles which will build to the goal of the macrocycle, we might suggest a preceding goal of a 10k in 6 months time. However, our runner has taken a couple of months off. So, In order to get on track for the 10k, which will ultimately determine if the athlete is on schedule for the future, our strategy might then involve the intermediate goal of a 5k run in 4 months time. Thus, our first few mesocycles will be directed towards the goal of the 5k.

To train optimally for the 5k, we would firstly understand that our primary aim would be VO$_2$max training, since the race involves working at a very high level for a reasonably short period of time. However, we would also understand that by training our athlete's metabolic fitness via LT work, he or she would be able to last longer at higher work rates by training to burn more fat and less carbohydrates overall, leading to a lower production of lactate. Thus, after a period of preparation, or "base work" of easy running which prepares the athlete to tolerate harder work later, we might consider starting the athlete on a significant amount of LT training. During this period, we would prescribe a small amount of VO$_2$ work, to prepare him/her for running faster and to again begin the process of adaptation to what will come later.

After the period of significant LT work, we would back off on the number of such workouts in favor of ramping up the more specific VO$_2$ work in preparation to race. Finally, in the last days before the race, we would reduce the overall training volume of our athlete, and perhaps conduct a very short taper in line with those we will discuss in the following chapter on tapering. The athlete should theoretically be in prime cardiovascular condition for the race, and hopefully the results would bear this out.

Part-way to our major goal race, we can now see the benefit of the reductionist view. In training over the first four months, the athlete was able to learn a great deal about how he or she felt in training, from the types of workouts/schedules that were too hard to the amount of improvement that was reasonable given their physiology. We can now decide the best way to peak for the 10k, and to have that protocol benefit the long term goal of the future half marathon. The athlete's oxygen transport system has now been maximized from the 5k training. These VO_2max workouts can now be reduced to "maintenance dose," and the athlete is free to perform LT work as the main race approaches, as LT would likely be more relevant to success at that distance than VO_2 alone, and still more relevant to the half-marathon distance. Furthermore, we know that improvements in LT can occur exclusive of improvements in VO_2max, a good thing since we decided that our athlete had gained the most possible out of the VO_2 system given the time allowed. In this case, these LT workouts could be designed based upon what the athlete felt worked best from the workouts done earlier in the season.

With the 10k out of the way, we would be able to make a decision. Is training going well, or is the athlete wiped out from training for a distance roughly half that of their macrocycle goal race. If the athlete is feeling run down, it might be to his or her advantage to put off the half-marathon in favor of backing off and taking some rest, and improving at the shorter distance of 10k, before making the step up. On the other hand, if the athlete was continuing to get stronger and was feeling well, we might consider reducing the VO_2 work to the bare minimum, and focusing on LT and more specific distance work in preparation for a coming half marathon.

You should understand that the above is a gross oversimplification on several levels. Firstly, workout distances and times would need to be specifically dictated, determined by the athlete and his or her strengths and weaknesses. Next, the particulars of those workouts would also be dictated by the goal race in terms of terrain, temperature, altitude, etc. Those points being made, we can see that it is possible to plan a training program using logical inference of physiologic principles. The fact that we do not have a garden of studies telling us the optimal training regimen is not a fatal flaw. It is up to the coach and athlete to discover/determine what the optimal periodization is through a personal experiment with just one subject: the athlete. To put it less glamorously, the process is to some extent trial and error. However, this process is something which will be incredibly illuminating to the athlete and lead to a great depth of understanding of their own personal physiology and athletic potential.

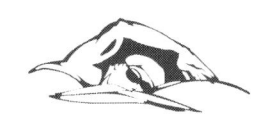

CHAPTER 8

Feeding the Machine

If you pick up any of the popular multisport or cycling magazines, you will see advertisements for every sort of supplement imaginable, from the ridiculous to the sublime. Before I start on what science tells us, I should make an important point: very, very few of the claims made by supplement manufacturers have ever been tested in an independent laboratory setting. Furthermore, even fewer have had such tests published in peer-reviewed scientific literature. In the United States, supplement manufacturers are not required to prove the efficacy of their products. Their claims do not undergo the extensive scrutiny of the Food and Drug administration. In fact, numerous studies have demonstrated that supplement manufacturers may put precious little of the supplement in question into their product. If you chemically analyzed ten commercial ginkgo tablets from different companies, you will almost certainly find huge differences in amount of the supposed active ingredients. You might also find a number of other chemicals, some of no benefit and some which could be outright dangerous.

> **Few supplements have ever been tested by an independent laboratory.**

You should be very wary of any manufacturer promising amazing performance gains with their new special brew formula, especially if you are not able to find any references to it in the scientific literature. Finding out if said great results have been reported by reputable scientists (rather than marketing hacks) is reasonably easy. Get on the Internet, and find your way to Pubmed. Pubmed is a free database of almost all the scientific literature in print. You will be able to look up papers by keyword, and you will usually be provided with a 250 word abstract, or blurb, about what the study was and what it did or did not show. For example, if some manufacturer had an ad out that showed that ingesting 8 oz. per day of their patented FastJuice (at $10/oz.) would increase your VO_2max by 33 percent, you go to Pubmed, type in FastJuice and VO_2, and see if anything pops up. Rest assured, if there was any credence to what most of these unscrupulous manufacturers was selling, it would almost immediately be published in *scientific* literature, probably because it would be a direct challenge to many years of established, tested science. Unfortunately, there is no free lunch.

Ultimately, my point is this: don't take marketing at face value. You are smarter than that. In fact, don't take my word either. Educate yourself. Get on Pubmed, read some of the abstracts, and if you find something interesting, order the whole paper and maybe a copy of a good physiology textbook. You can figure this stuff out, and decide for yourself if someone is legitimate or if they are selling hair tonic.

There are a few ways to improve your athletic performance. We have discussed training. You could have selected parents who were more gifted physiologically, but there is no re-choosing on that front. Or, as you might imagine, you can optimize what goes into your body. It's the fuel that runs your engine, and there is no sense cutting the gas with water, so to speak. Honestly, an appropriate training diet is beyond the scope of this work, but I will try to provide you with some basic guidelines to help point you in the right direction.

Diet

What do I eat before I race or train?
The bad news is that everyone has a different opinion with respect to this. The *good* news is that they are all correct. Allow me to explain. For years, people have argued over what the pre-race meal ought to consist of. There have been well-replicated experiments that show that low glycemic index foods (i.e. foods that don't hit you with a huge rush of simple sugar: think of an apple vs. a candy bar) allow greater liberation of fat into the bloodstream with exercise. Other studies showed that high glycemic index carbohydrates in the 30 min before exercise might impair performance. Still other studies showed that a large amount of carbohydrates right before exercise actually enhance and improve performance.

A good study by Burke and colleagues in 1998, which was run under conditions similar to racing, showed that so long as you are consuming an appropriate carbohydrate/electrolyte drink (i.e. Gatorade) at appropriate time intervals, it really does not matter what you ate before the race.[52] They fed people either high or low glycemic index carbohydrates, or a control meal with almost no carbohydrates before testing them on a cycle ergometer. While riding, they had the athlete's drink a carbohydrate drink, which most of us would do. After 20 minutes, there was no difference in the amount of fat in their bloodstream. Nor was there any difference in the amount of glucose in their blood. In other words, drinking the sports drink cancelled out the effects of the pre-race meal. Intuitively, this makes sense. Whatever was going on in your body after you ate is going to be radically changed when you start exercising and start slugging down a sweet drink, which is certainly going to raise the amount of carbohydrates entering your blood stream. The take home message is that you should eat what you are comfortable eating before a race, and more importantly what you have found works for you in the past.

What to consume during exercise

This subject has been studied ad nauseum. The consensus from the literature for quite some time has been that you should consume approximately 1 gram per minute/1-1.2 g/kg/hour of carbohydrates. The studies in question used various carbohydrates, although it was often just glucose. However, there were some interesting results from a recent paper by Roy et al.[53] You have multiple mechanisms for transporting carbohydrates from your intestines to your blood. In fact, you have transporters specific to different types of carbohydrates. What these guys did was use a mixed beverage that contained glucose, fructose, and sucrose. Their thought was that these would each be transported by a separate mechanism, leading to an even higher concentration in the blood.

This is exactly what the study showed. Utilizing the mixed beverage and consuming roughly 2.4 g/min, participants were able to achieve oxidation rates of 1.7 g/minute. This allowed the participants to use a higher amount of ingested carbohydrate for energy, and thus use less of their stored carbohydrates (glycogen). These data would seem to lend support to the practice of those athletes who consume varying foodstuffs during exercise. Since the multiple sugars are entering the body via different transporters, they are theoretically sparing their internal energy stores and are able to go longer before fatigue.

My recommendation would be to experiment a bit and see what works for you. Use varying carbohydrates in different mixtures in either liquid (sports drink) or liquid and solid form (gels, bars, or regular food). Your goal is to eat and drink a combination that does not upset your stomach while training or racing. There is no need to get much above 2 grams/minute. It might not hurt, but it is likely more than your body is able to use. Of course, any extra you consume remains in your gut and may serve to help maintain the carbohydrate flow into your body during periods when you cannot eat or drink enough.

There is also the important subject of gastric emptying, or the rate at which fluid is moved from your stomach into your intestines. The general rule of thumb is that the more concentrated the solution, the more slowly it empties from the stomach. Also, liquids are emptied more quickly than solids.[54] This means a couple of things. Firstly, water will empty from the stomach quickly, and in fact a sports drink of 6-8% carbohydrate will empty at the same rate. As you increase the concentration, emptying is slowed. This is not necessarily important in terms of caloric delivery, because although the stomach empties more slowly, each bit emptied contains more calories. It is important, however, in that it leads to the stomach becoming distended, leading to a feeling of fullness and the possibility of nausea. The bottom line is that you will need to experiment in order to find the optimum recipe for getting enough calories into your body without getting an upset stomach.

What do I eat after I race or train?
This is another good question. There are lots of supplement manufacturers out there telling you to drink their recovery drink, because it has protein or fat or amino acids in it that will improve recovery, whatever that means. (Presumably, we are talking about restocking your body's stores of carbohydrates post-exercise, but we don't know what those marketing people are talking about.) So let's look at this more closely.

There are, in fact, studies which seem to show that eating carbohydrates with protein post-exercise causes quicker restocking of the muscles with glycogen. Zawadski and colleagues showed in 1992 that protein and carbohydrates consumed post exercise did exactly that.[55] Tarnopolsky and colleagues showed, in 1997, that a carbohydrate/protein/fat solution post exercise also increase muscle glycogen, but not significantly differently than carbohydrate alone.[56] These studies also showed an increase in plasma insulin levels, which is the hormone your body uses to help push carbohydrate into your cells to make glycogen. Certain manufacturers have made claims that it is this increase in insulin with added protein or protein plus fat that makes the difference, thus making you recover faster. Well, does it?

Firstly, the Zawadski study was flawed to begin with. If you are going to claim that the composition of two meals (namely, carbohydrate or carbohydrate plus protein) makes a difference, you need to make sure that all other aspects of those meals are the same. In other words, there should be equivalent calories in each. In that study, there were 39% more calories in the carbohydrate + protein meal. Furthermore, an excellent study by Jentgens et al made the excellent observation that insulin was *not* the limiting factor in getting more glycogen made quicker. In other words, you need relatively little insulin to get your carbohydrate transporters working full-blast, so more is not necessarily better. So, you don't need any fancy drinks with special formulae to get recovered. You need about 1.2 grams of carbohydrate per kilogram of your body weight per hour, and you need to be eating around every half hour for the couple hours immediately post exercise.[57] (This is obviously more important if you are racing or training multiple times a day and need to be back in full working order quickly.)

"Okay," You say, "So I should eat all carbohydrates post exercise, right?" Wrong. Your exercise damaged your body. You broke down some muscle and connective tissue. Those things need to be repaired, and one of the materials used is protein. Furthermore, you need fat in your diet. It is what is used to make the membranes that hold your cells together, among other things. So we are back to the old standby…you need to eat a balanced diet. Lean meats, grains, dairy and an appropriate amount of fat all have their place in a healthy person's diet. Anytime someone suggests some new fantastic supplement or diet plan, go to the nearest mirror and open your mouth. You will see teeth. In fact, you will see a few different kinds. You have incisors and canines for grasping and cutting meat, and you have molars for grinding grains and legumes. Those choppers were developed by Mother Nature over millions of years for those purposes. If you were meant to suck down special concoctions, you would have been provided with a built in straw instead of teeth. If you were meant to eat all meat, you'd have more canine teeth and you'd look like your dog. If you were meant to eat all vegetable matter, you'd have a mouth like a cow: almost all molars. You are an omnivore: you were built to eat everything. Don't fight Mother Nature.

> **You are an omnivore.**
> Don't fight Mother Nature.

Low Carbohydrate vs. High carbohydrate
Forget the Atkins Cult. Erase the low-carbohydrate craze from your mind. You are an athlete now and your body is screaming for carbohydrates when you exercise. A diet low in carbohydrates has been show in innumerable studies to decrease time to fatigue, and decrease the amount of athletic work you can perform. One source of fatigue is when your muscles run out of glycogen, which is your body's storage form of carbohydrate. After exercise, your muscles are hungry for carbohydrates. They want to fill the tank back up. If you limit your carbohydrates, you never replenish your stores and your body is running sub-optimally. Again, exercise burns quite a bit of fat when done often and in sufficient length, however, your body is almost always burning a mixture of fat and carbohydrate. With endurance training, your body will learn to burn a higher percentage of fat to meet your energy needs, and use relatively less carbohydrates, but it will always and without fail use both in any race longer than a few minutes.

> **A diet low** in carbohydrates will decrease time to fatigue.

What about carbohydrate loading? It is possible to run down your glycogen stores leading up to a race by limiting carbohydrate intake and continuing to exercise, followed by eating a lot of pasta the day or two before the race. There is some scientific backing for this methodology, and you can indeed follow such a protocol to maximize the amount of carbohydrates loaded into your muscles before the race. However, I do not believe that the difference between such a protocol and simply maximizing your carbohydrate intake in the days leading up to your big race is worthwhile. In general, athletes who follow the carbohydrate loading protocols feel terrible in the time they are limiting themselves. (Ask your friends how they felt when they started on the Atkins' diet. You will feel worse because of the amount of exercise you will be attempting when under fueled.) I do not feel that this is psychologically beneficial to the athlete. You want to feel strong and powerful as you approach race day, not shaky from a sudden change in diet.

Interestingly, dietary manipulation along these lines will apparently increase the amount of fat your body will burn. In a study by Carey and colleagues back in 2001, long distance cyclists were fed a fat rich, carbohydrate depleted diet for about a week.[61] They continued training, and at the end of the "dietary intervention," they were rested a day and then stuffed with carbohydrates for a day. Then they were sent out on a four hour bike ride, followed by a 1 hour time trial. When compared with cyclists who had not been given a high fat diet, these cyclists burned relatively more fat, thus sparing glycogen. More importantly, the fat-eating cyclists had an 11% increase in their TT power output, corresponding to an overall improvement in performance of about 4%.

It should be noted that this improvement was not statistically significant, mostly because there were not enough persons in this study to reliably detect a change of 4%. Had there been more participants, the result might have reached "significance," or not. The authors comment that in an ultra distance event (i.e. Ironman) a difference of even a couple percent is major, and might mean the difference between qualifying for the world championships or a podium spot and going home thinking "if only I could have shaved a few more minutes off of my bike time at the end." I'm certainly not suggesting that you go all fat and no carbohydrates, for the reasons I mentioned previously, but it stands to reason that you should at least maintain your fat intake in the run up to a race, especially since limiting fat seems to have the side effect of decreasing the amount of fat that you burn.

It should also be noted that if you are continually drinking a carbohydrate replacement beverage, you will also be burning those carbohydrates and will hopefully go a lot longer before wholly tapping out your glycogen reserves. Again, you should be consuming around 1 to 1.2 grams of carbohydrate per kilogram of your body weight per hour, or about a gram a minute.[62] (If you believe the Roy et al study, you can bump that up to around 2 grams of a mixed carbohydrate peparation). But what if your plans go awry on race day? What if your stomach gets upset and you can't keep up with what you should be eating and drinking? You can look at the aforementioned study as a little insurance. By burning less glycogen and more fat, you are ensuring that you have a little extra in the tank if you have a problem getting enough carbohydrates into your body, meaning you have more time to get straightened out before you bonk. It is food for thought, anyway.

Hydration
There are multiple sources on the Internet and in print telling you to ingest varying amounts of fluid during exercise. I have had multiple athletes tell me that they were instructed by coaches to stay far ahead of their thirst; that if they ever actually felt thirsty, it was too late and they were behind on their fluids. I'm going to tell you that drinking to thirst is almost exactly what you ought to be doing. In fact, if you are drinking more than about a liter or so per hour you are risking a condition known as hyponatremia, or low blood sodium.

Hyponatremia (with regard to exercise, anyway) is a condition in which you ingest too much fluid, which dilutes the amount of salt in your bloodstream.[59] It has been suggested that the salt in sports drink will prevent hyponatremia if you drink enough. This is false. The amount of salt in sports drinks is below the concentration of salt in your bodily fluids, thus it will only serve to dilute the salt in your body. It has also been suggested that taking salt tablets will improve the situation by replacing lost salt, thus preventing hyponatremia. A study by Speedy et al in 2002 showed that this is also a misconception[59]. Again, the problem with hyponatremia is low salt due to dilution, not low salt because you have actually lost salt (although you do lose a little). Your kidneys are, in fact, very good at conserving salt. Moreover, most people do not lose much salt through sweat, as your body has mechanisms to recover much of the salt that would otherwise be in your sweat.

The only reason you might consider using salt tablets is that Speedy showed that they seem to decrease weight loss during ultra-distance exercise, indicating that the athletes who supplement with the tablets lose slightly less fluid due to the salt. However, I doubt this effect is significant enough to warrant their use. My advice would be to save the money, to drink appropriately, and let your body take care of the sodium issue.

Why do we want to avoid hyponatremia? Without getting too far into the subtleties of how your body handles fluids and electrolytes, let me put it this way: mild hyponatremia may leave you feeling queasy, moderate hyponatremia will almost certainly send you to the medical tent, and severe hyponatremia will cause swelling of your brain, seizures, and possibly death. Please, please don't over drink. Keep it under about a liter per hour and drink when you are thirsty.

Supplements

The Placebo Effect

I think any discussion of supplements should begin here. A placebo is something that has no effect, good or bad, which we give to experimental subjects as a comparison to those subjects who have received something whose effects we want to test. For example, if we wanted to find out if my new supplement FastJuice helped performance, we would give half of our test subjects FastJuice and the other half a placebo (for example, a sugar pill). Then we would test our subjects and see if the FastJuice group performed significantly better than the sugar pill group.

The above experiment only works if the subjects (and to be strict, the testers) are unaware of which people got the supplement and which got the sugar pill. To do otherwise opens our experiment to what is known as the placebo effect. You can think of this as "mind over matter." In other words, the power of suggestion is a powerful thing, and the believing mind can coerce spectacular things from the willing body.

An example of this can be found in a 1972 study by Ariel and colleagues.[60] Basically, they took a group of weight lifters on a strength program and followed their progress. In 7 weeks, the athletes improved their maximal lift by about 2 percent. They then began injecting some of them with a placebo which the lifters believed was an anabolic steroid. In just 4 weeks, the lifters improved their maximal lift by about 10%. The only explanation (other than that the placebo was switched for real steroids) is that the subjects minds were able to alter their physical states.

The take home message is that when you are evaluating a study which a manufacturer claims shows a benefit; you should look for a couple of things. You should make sure that there is a placebo group and there is a group receiving the supplement in question. You should make sure that the study is double blind, meaning that neither the subject nor the experimenter knew who was getting the supplement and who was getting the placebo. Finally, you should hopefully make sure the groups are age and gender matched. You should not accept that a study done on eighty year old women applied to teenage boys.

Hi-test vs. Decaf

Visit the Internet discussion lists and you will often see the question: does caffeine help athletic performance? The short answer is yes. However, the story is a little more complicated than that, and there are some things you need to know if you are hoping that your addiction to Fourbucks is going to help your times on race day. (It might not.)

Okay, first of all, does it work? Yes, according to Kovacs and colleagues, who studied the question in 1998.[63] Well trained cyclists and triathletes who were supplemented with 150, 225, and 320 mg/L of caffeine all improved their performance in a 1 hour time trial versus those who received water alone, or water plus carbohydrate. Those who received water completed the TT in 62.5 min, those who received 150 mg/L caffeine solution took 60.4 min, and those who took the 225 or 320 completed it in 58.9 minutes. During and after the time trial, athletes who had consumed caffeine had higher blood levels of lactate, which probably reflects the higher amount of work they were able to do while using caffeine. Interestingly, there was no performance benefit in going from 225 mg/L to 320 mg/L.

This study also answered another important question: will caffeine get me banned from sports with a positive urine test? In this study, all persons taking caffeine had urine levels lower than those set by the anti-doping authorities of the IOC. However, the authors recommend a dose of 4.5 mg/kg body weight to ensure compliance. This question will be slightly less relevant after 2004, because caffeine will be removed from the WADA banned list in 2005.

"Great." You are saying, "But my daily cup of Fourbucks makes me pee like a racehorse. I'm not going to be going any faster if I have to pull over to water the plants. Not to mention I'll get dehydrated, which will slow me down big time." I have good news. This study and others also indicate that:

1. Exercise counteracts the diuretic effect that caffeine has on people at rest.
2. Caffeine does not increase body temperature or sweat volume during exercise.
3. Caffeine does not decrease blood plasma volume.

Now, we come to the caveats. Firstly, Bell and colleagues in

2002 showed that there is a much greater increase in performance in athletes who are *not* regular caffeine users.[64] Also, it appeared that caffeine's effects lasted at least 6 hours in non-users, and somewhat less in users. Time to exhaustion is greater when you give caffeine to those who are not regular caffeine users. So, you are going to have to break your coffee habit if you want to see the maximum benefit.

The next problem is that it seems like you can't just drink a bunch of coffee on race day; the best results are seen with a caffeine supplement, *not* just plain coffee. They postulate that there are other compounds in the coffee that might counteract the performance enhancing effect. Also, caffeine probably won't help you burn fat, or spare glycogen, for that matter, no matter what the supplement manufacturers want to tell you. Finally, caffeine can cause anxiety, nausea, and dizziness. None of these will help your performance. In other words, moderation in everything, and don't try this for the first time before your A-race.

Another important point is that caffeine seems to have beneficial effects when taken during exercise. A study by Van Nieuwenhoven and colleagues looked at water vs. carbohydrate/electrolyte solution (i.e. Gatorade) vs. the same solution with 150 mg/L caffeine.[65] They were trying to answer several questions, most importantly what would the effect be on the GI tract. What they found was that the caffeinated solution significantly increased the absorption of glucose from the intestine. Also, they found that the caffeine did not cause reflux (the phenomena that causes heartburn and associated belching), a change in acidity in the stomach (which may or may not be associated with an upset stomach), or gastrointestinal transit time (i.e. diarrhea or constipation). However, I am not suggesting that you load up on caffeine throughout your Ironman race. This test was run on a cycle ergometer for 90 minutes. In other words, none of the above caused a problem in over a short time period, along the lines of a sprint race. What would happen over a longer period of time, or with more caffeine, is anyone's guess. Again, my point is that you should not try anything on race day that you did not try in training. You aren't going to be any faster if you are stopping to hit the porta-john's every ten miles.

Medium Chain Triglycerides: run faster, or get the trots?
MCT's are fat. However, this particular fat is liquid at room temperature. For a time, it was thought that it would be of benefit during exercise because it is very quickly broken down and absorbed by the body. Medium chain triglycerides are more soluble in water, and apparently empty from the stomach better than the equivalent calorie sports drink. In theory, this is all good stuff. However, numerous studies have shown that taking a dose of the stuff before submaximal *or* high intensity exercise does not lengthen time to exhaustion, or help you burn any more fat than you would if you were just drinking a sports drink alone. Furthermore, a study by Angus et al in 2000 compared a placebo drink (water with no-calorie sweetener) with sports drink or sports drink + MCT's in a 100km TT.[66] They found that while the sports drink improved performance more than the placebo, no additional benefit was gained by adding the MCT's.

One particularly unwanted side effect of MCT's is stomach distress. People who were fed around 30 grams of the stuff reported cramping, discomfort, and diarrhea. Once again, we are talking about an important question of risk versus benefit. The possible benefit is going faster; however, the aforementioned study seems to contradict this. The very definite risk is that you will end up defecating behind someone's bushes at the roadside because you gave yourself diarrhea. And that will make you *much* slower, especially if the owner calls the cops and has you arrested. Will the cops tow an expensive time trial bike, or just put it half in/half out of their trunk so that the lid can bounce up and down on the nice paint job all the way to the station? I don't know, and you don't want to find out.

Creatine: It works, but not for you

A couple of years ago, creatine was all the rage. It is still being used, but not quite as extensively, at least not in the patients I have seen. The short version is that it does, in fact, seem to have some effect in power sports, for example, weight lifting. It is of much less use to an endurance athlete. Allow me to explain.

Earlier in the book, we discussed how your body makes energy, and how that energy is stored in the form of ATP. If you start exercising intensely, you start breaking down your ATP very quickly. It takes a short time to ramp up production. In the meantime, you have something in your muscle cells called Creatine Phosphate. This chemical serves to regenerate the ATP in the short term. All well and good, however, you run down this chemical in about ten seconds.[67] So it would stand to reason that if you could store more of this Creatine Phosphate, you could regenerate more ATP for longer. It should also stand to reason that extra creatine should only be useful under conditions where you are using a *lot* of ATP in a *very* short time.

You normally have about 125 mmol of Cr per kilogram of muscle mass. In a number of studies, participants have been able to increase their stores a maximum of another 20% or so with supplementation. However, this was not possible with diet. Raw meat contains 4-5 grams creatine per kg, and cooking breaks some of that down.[68] Suffice it to say you can't eat enough, so you would have to buy a supplement.

Okay, so we believe that we can indeed increase the amount of creatine in our muscles. Do we believe it can increase performance? Yes. In one study, time to exhaustion during intense exercise increased from 118 to 154 seconds.[69] In another study, it was observed to increase one-rep maximum bench press, vertical jump performance, and decrease 100 yd sprint times. In another test series of 300 meter and 1000 meter sprints, it was shown to reduce the times on average by about 0.3 seconds in the 300 and by 2.1 seconds in the 1000.[70]

The question you must ask yourself is what relevance this has to the endurance athlete? Well, when you race, does it take shorter or longer than 154 seconds? It is a little more complicated than that, but you get my meaning. Creatine is something that could help you if you raced over a very short distance, going all out, and then only by a little bit. It has not been shown to be of help in distances longer than around 1000 meters.

What about the down sides? When taken during exercise, creatine has been shown to cause post-exercise distress and syncope ("passing out"), so don't do that. Also, it appears to cause a significant weight gain of 1-5 kg, presumably because of increased water retention. That is a serious problem. Remember when we talked about the concept of power to weight ratio? If we raise your weight, but don't raise your VO_2, then we have made you slower. As there is no evidence that Creatine raises your $V0_2$, but there is a lot of evidence that creatine raises your body weight, it is tough to justify it's use in an endurance athlete.

Branched Chain Amino Acids
Amino acids are the building blocks of proteins. Your body can synthesize many of them, and some must be provided in your diet. There are 21 different amino acids, each of which has a different chemical structure. Some of them are a single chain of carbon, nitrogen, hydrogen and nitrogen atoms, and others have branch points or even ring structures. Branched chain amino acids (BCAA's) include valine, leucine and isoleucine. They have been touted as ergogenic, and endurance aids by supplement manufacturers. There is little evidence supporting this.

Minerals
Many dietary and sports supplements claim that the addition of trace minerals have ergogenic benefits. For example, chromium has been claimed to cause increases in lean muscle mass by aiding insulin action. It has also been claimed to have a direct ergogenic effect. Unfortunately, there have been no good studies I have been able to find which support these claims. Moreover, the FDA has

actually requested that manufacturers stop making false claims about the benefits of chromium.

The story is similar with other trace elements, such as vanadium and zinc. These metals might find an appropriate place in your bicycle frame, however, there is really no evidence that any amount greater than that naturally found in food is of any benefit. My opinion would be to avoid these preparations and save your money for something that really will do you some good in a race, like healthy breakfast.

Herbs

Two herbs (*Cordyceps sinensis* and *Rhodiola rosea*) have gained press over the years for their purported ability to alter VO$_2$ kinetics. They are currently sold in the United States under the brand name Optygen by First Endurance. A study by Earnest et al published in March 2004 showed no positive benefit in endurance cycling performance.[71]

Illegal Performance Enhancing Agents

In terms of increasing endurance capacity, there is really only one way to do it unnaturally: increasing the fraction of red blood cells that your heart is pumping at any given time. This has been done a couple of ways. You could give yourself a transfusion of blood, which instantly increases your blood volume and the fraction of total blood that is carrying oxygen. This is called blood doping, and was the reason that dishonor was brought to US Cycling in the early 80's. It is also very dangerous. Another way of doing this is by taking EPO (erythropoietin, sold under several brand names). This is a substance normally produced by your kidneys that causes your body to produce more red blood cells. Again, this will increase the amount of exercise you can do because your muscles will receive more oxygen per heart beat. Once again, you are taking your life in your hands. A case report in the journal Neurology described an elite cyclist who developed a blood clot in the brain because of "sludging".[72] Basically, all the extra red blood cells in your vessels begin to hang up in certain places, like mud in the bends of a river. This is probably exacerbated by dehydration during exercise, which could make the blood more viscous. It is only a matter of time before something gets plugged up and you risk a major stroke or heart attack. Do you like your pizza by the slice, or ground into a thin paste and fed to you through a tube after you have a stroke and cannot eat by mouth? I am being a little dramatic, but this is the chance you are taking. The question you must ask yourself is how much that cheesy age-group trophy is worth to you.

You could probably safely use EPO under the careful supervision of a physician, if you maintained proper hydration at all times and had regular blood tests. In fact, I have many patients who are on chemotherapy for cancer or who have kidney failure and require it to lead a normal life. However, it is cheating in the realm of sports. Moreover, we do not necessarily know the long term health effects of chronically ramping up your production of red blood cells. As with all things, you will have to decide what you can live with, and again what you are willing to risk for the dubious goal of a race win.

Ephedra/Pseudoephedrine

The question as to whether ephedra is ergogenic or not is moot at this point, as supplements containing it have recently been banned in the United States. In my medical opinion, this is a good thing, as in recent years I have seen numerous patients admitted to the hospital with dangerous heart rhythms as a direct result of ephedra ingestion. I would never recommend or condone an athlete risking their health by taking it. Pseudoephedrine has similar effects to ephedra. At the time of this writing, it is also banned in competition.

That being said, it seems that ephedra works. Jacobs and coworkers published a paper in 2003 showing that ephedra (0.8 mg/kg), or a combination of ephedra and caffeine (4mg/kg) significantly improved participants leg press repetitions versus placebo (average repetitions 16 and 19 respectively, vs. 13 for placebo).[73] It should be noted, however, that performance was only increased during the first set. The authors concluded that the effect was largely due to the ephedra. Other studies, notably Bell et al showed that ephedra + caffeine significantly decreased 10k run times, and that this effect was largely seen in the last 5 km of the run.[74] This study also concluded that the effect was largely due to the ephedra, and that there was no additive effect with caffeine.

> **Ephedra** can cause heart rhythm disturbances.

Let me reiterate: you'll be a little faster on ephedra. You'll be a lot slower if you drop dead from a heart arrhythmia. Think carefully before you risk your health or life.

CHAPTER 9

Tapering To Race

Athletes often discuss their taper before a race, and they are usually quite nervous about it. Essentially, what they are talking about is a reduction in training intensity or duration (or both) in the time immediately leading up to a race, so that they recover completely from training, and get stronger in time to have their best possible performance on race day. If you want the official scientific definition, Neary and co-workers call it a training technique designed to "reverse training induced fatigue without a loss of the training adaptations."[75]

Most of us generally "feel" better after backing off of heavy training for a couple of days, but is there any objective research suggesting that it is to our advantage? If so, how should we design our taper? These are the issues I would like to examine today. In fact, there have been a number of good studies addressing the question of the taper. The short answer to the question, "Will a taper make me faster on race day?" is yes, provided that it is done right.

One particularly straightforward study that looked both at simulated race times and the biochemical changes resulting from tapering was carried out by Neary et al in 2003.[76] Neary set up three groups of cyclists who were similar in their physiologic makeup. He put them all on the same exercise program for 7 weeks, which consisted of 60 minutes/day, 4 days per week at 85-90% of their maximum heart rate. In the final week of training, he had one group continue training the same, one group continue the same amount of training but with progressively less intensity each day (85% HRmax, then 75%, 65%, 55% respectively), and another group keep up their intensity but reduce the total amount of training each day (45', 35',25', 20'). They were tested with simulated 40K TT performances before and after the taper programs. Afterwards, they had samples taken from their muscles and analyzed for the amount of different enzymes as well as what type of muscle fibers these enzymes were found in.

As it turned out, the group that maintained intensity of training but reduced time improved their 40k TT by 4.3%, while there was no change in the other two groups. VO$_2$max was also increased slightly in that group, but not in the other two. Finally, power output at ventilatory threshold increased in both taper groups, but was greater in the group that maintained intensity (12%) vs. the group that maintained duration of exercise (8%). Neary and his group attribute most of the positive adaptations to increases in oxidative enzymes, increased contractility, as well as maintenance of the total volume of muscle mass primarily in the Type IIa fibers (The fast-twitch, oxidative fibers).

> **A taper** maintaining intensity but reducing exercise time will improve race performance

Similar findings have also been noted in swimmers. Trappe et al looked at the effect of taper on whole muscles and on individual fibers after a 21 day taper.[77] However, in this taper protocol, duration was decreased and intensity was increased in an effort to mimic race paces. At the end of the taper, swim power was measured by a tether device attached to the swimmer. They found a 13% increase in power, and a 4% improvement in race time. When they looked at the peak force of individual muscle cells, they found that the Type IIa fibers went up by 30%. However, muscle fiber size had also increased, and this probably accounts for the difference. The contractile speed went up by 32% in the type I (slow twitch) fibers and by 67% in the type IIa fibers. Thus, the improvement in the type IIa fibers was much greater than that in the type I (in fact, the increased contractile speed was the only improvement seen in the type I fibers). Finally, muscle fiber size increased in the type IIa fibers by 11%.

Fiber types aside, the point I am trying to make is that the benefit of the taper is actually physiologic, and not just psychological. There are genuine, measurable changes in biochemistry and force production that will give you an edge over the athlete that trained right up until race day, or the one who rested too much. Though you might find yourself a little nervous by "slacking" in the days leading up to your big race, console yourself with the knowledge that your body is recovering and you are getting stronger, not weaker by backing off. But are there other beneficial changes?

> **The benefit** of the taper is physiologic and not just psychological

It has been shown that the taper causes improvements in blood characteristics. This was recently looked at by Mujika in 2000, who studied middle distance runners.[78] The runners performed 15 weeks of training, and then either did a moderate or low volume taper, while maintaining their interval work. He asked the runners to perform a couple of 800M runs before the taper protocol and after. The results indicated an increase in production of red blood cells, as well as plasma expansion, both of which would serve to improve performance through an increase in VO$_2$max, although this study in particular did not show that.

Other studies have shown more dramatically that the taper seems to be effective for distance runners. A good representative study was done by Houmard et al in 1994.[79] By maintaining interval training and reducing volume by 85%, runners reduced their times by 3% in a 5k at self selected pace. They also had a significant decrease (6%) in their submaximal oxygen consumption, indicating an improvement in economy. This is in line with most studies reviewed by Mujika in 2003, who indicated that in general tapering athletes improve their performance between 0.5% and

6%.[80]

Finally, there have been studies that show taper protocols are beneficial to triathletes in particular, and not just single sport athletes. Banister et al studied the difference between a stepwise taper (that is, a step off in the amount of training to some percentage less) and an exponential taper in 1999.[82] They found that the exponential 5 day taper group cycled better, and ran better (though not significantly so) in the 5k run than the stepwise taper of equivalent duration. Also, faster tapers (4 days) performed better in maximal cycling tests and again ran better (again, not significantly so) in a 5k.

The most difficult question to answer is regarding the optimal length of taper. Unfortunately, I cannot provide you with a recipe. About the most specific study I have found was conducted by Kenitzer in 1998[82], who concluded that 2 weeks was the cutoff between recovery and the beginnings of detraining. (His protocol involved blood lactate measurements and recorded performance times of a standardized workout among a group of female swimmers). I cite that study because swimmers are notorious for training volumes far above race distance, much like high level Iron-distance triathletes. Dr. Timothy Noakes of the University of Cape Town S.A. also had a paper out of his lab suggesting that athletes who train particularly long hours also required roughly 2 weeks of recovery to maximize their adaptations.[83]

Please remember that numerous studies have suggested other

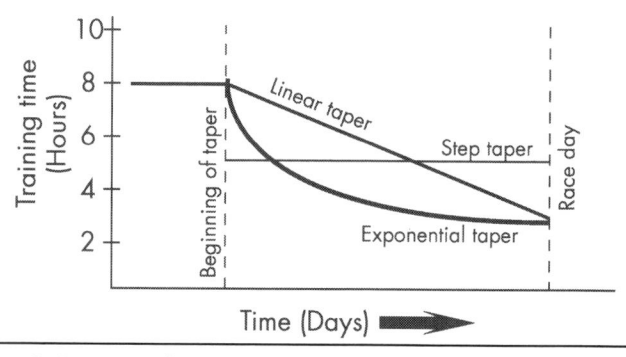

Figure 9.0   A schematic representation of different tapering strategies.

optimal lengths ranging from a couple of days to almost a month, with many in the middle. This would indicate to me that the taper length is very specific to the individual, and falls more in the realm of coaching art than it does exercise science, at least at this time. My educated opinion would be that you should do a longer 2 week taper for Iron events, and a shorter taper for shorter events. You could certainly argue me on that point and I would not dispute you. I would certainly advise some experimentation to find out what works best for you (figure 9.0).

If you have access to a university library, I highly recommend Mujika's 2003 article on the many different types of tapers[80]. In fact, I would almost consider it required reading for those of you interested in learning more about, and designing your own taper. It reviews most of the recent articles on the subject, and serves to compare the differing taper formats and their relative performance benefits. The take home message from his analysis is that it is important to maintain intensity, to reduce volume between 60 and 90%, and perhaps reduce frequency slightly in the run up to your big race. Finally, you are better off with a progressive, nonlinear taper (i.e. an exponential curve), than you are with a simple step-wise reduction.

CHAPTER 10

Race Day

Race day is the fruition of your training. It is the day you can finally let loose and see what you are capable of. That said, there are a few keys that will help you execute your plan as smoothly possible.

Warm-up

We all do a warm up of some kind: jogging around the parking lot, swimming a few strokes to make sure our goggles are on right, or zipping up the road on the bike to make sure everything is functioning well and we will start out in the right gear. When I have asked fellow athletes why they do the warm up, I noted the following responses:

"It helps me relax before the gun."
"It makes me confident that my gear is in working order."
"It gets me loose."

Psychological reasons aside, there actually have been a few studies on the effect of different warm-ups on measurable physiologic parameters. In 1991, Houmard et al looked at a group of college swimmers whose task was to do a 365 meter swim at around 95% of their VO_2max. 5 minutes after warm-up.[84] One trial was done without warm-up, one with a warm-ups with 4 x

50M hard on 1 minute rest, one with a medium intensity warm-up (65% of VO_2max), and one that combined the high intensity and medium intensity warm-ups.

As it turned out, the no-warm-up trial caused a shorter stroke distance in the last 100M, and significantly higher levels of lactate post exercise when compared with the medium or medium + intervals warm-ups. Heart rate post exercise was also significantly higher when there as no warm-up. Interestingly, the high intensity warm-up alone was no better than skipping the warm-up entirely. Finally, there was no difference at all between the medium warm-up and the medium plus intervals warm-up.

These data would seem to suggest that the longer, medium paced swim is going to give you the most bang for your buck in terms of a warm-up. However, it also seems clear that you could throw a few intervals in there and it would not hurt very much.

> **A long, medium paced warm-up may be most beneficial.**

Personally, I feel that it isn't wise to expend too much energy pre-race, but I cannot deny that I feel better while racing after I have spent a minute or two at my race pace before I go out there for real. It helps me remember how fast I want to go, and what my overall plan is. Your mileage may vary, as they say. In other words, experiment and see what works for you.

Stretching

After a warm-up, and before training or racing, many athletes perform stretching. There was an excellent review paper published in March 2004 by Thacker et al which looked at much of the published literature on the subject of stretching on sports injury.[85] The authors cite multiple studies which do not show a correlation between increased flexibility or stretching and decreased risk of injury. Also, their analysis indicates an increase in risk of injury with an excessive amount of flexibility.

Firstly, does stretching in fact increase the range of motion of joints? Yes. In general, stretching seems to result increase flexibility for up to 90 minutes.[86] (That being said, my clinical experience seems to suggest a slightly shorter time course, of perhaps an hour or so). Also, stretching programs over the course of weeks have been shown to increase flexibility for several weeks afterwards.[87]

In my review of the available literature, I found very few honestly good papers. Many are serviceable, and can give us some idea, but overall I was unable to find a truly definitive analysis. The above review seems to be the closest thing available to an objective analysis across the board, and their conclusion is similar to mine: i.e. you really cannot endorse or deny the benefits of stretching based on current research.

Based on my clinical experience, and that of many good sports physicians I have worked with, I would give the following advice: stretching, when done in order to correct a biomechanical imbalance, is probably safe and effective. However, your goal is *not* to increase flexibility to the maximal amount you can. Your goal is to attain full physiologic range of motion. In other words, to allow your joint to work fully in the angles it is meant to. By overstretching, you are simply decreasing the amount that your soft tissues are able to prevent joint injury by reducing unnatural motion in that joint. If you are *not* having problems with injury due to imbalances of strength/flexibility (i.e. patellofemoral syndrome), and do *not* feel tight in the natural ranges of motion you experience in your sport, there is no reason to spend a great deal of time working on flexibility. If a little stretch makes you feel better before you work out or race, fine. Just be smart and don't over do it.

Pace and strategy

A long time ago, there was a John Cusack movie called, "Better Off Dead." In the course of the film, he challenges the local ski-stud to a race down the K12, the "gnarliest run in town." On a practice run, he stands atop the mountain with his best friend, Charles DeMar, who gives him the following advice. "Go that way. Really fast. If something gets in your way, turn."

CHAPTER 10
Race Day

If only it were that easy. In the real world, you need to use your head as much as your legs. There has been quite a bit of work done on the finer points of getting from A to B using the muscle between your ears.

First things first: no one has yet been able to associate swim performance with overall triathlon performance.[88] Our experience bears this out: we all have friends who are stellar swimmers, who come out in the front of the pack as they exit the water and slowly fall behind throughout the rest of the race. Alternatively, we are all familiar with the results of the 2001 Ironman Lake Placid, in which professional cyclist Steve Larsen exited the water in the middle of the pack…of the amateurs, that is, not the professionals! He then proceeded to set the Lake Placid bike course record and go on to win the race. Your goal is not to win the swim; it is to lose no more time than you can make up with your bike and run talents. If you happen to be a particularly talented swimmer and can put a little time into your competition, there is nothing wrong with that. The point is not to kill yourself trying to build an insurmountable lead. It doesn't work.

What about drafting? Nearly all races are draft legal on the swim. You are wasting precious energy if you aren't sitting on the heels of someone who is going around the speed you want to be going. According to a study by Chartard et al in 1998, drafting allows the training swimmer to take advantage of a decreased pressure gradient.[89] In other words, the front swimmer must "break through" the pressure he or she encounters by pushing through unbroken water, and the trailer takes advantage of this. The trailing swimmer encounters between 10% and 26% less drag using this strategy. The effect of drafting is highlighted by a 10% decrease in oxygen uptake, a 6.2% decrease in HR, and an 11-31% decrease in lactate concentration. The best position was somewhere between 0 and 50 cm behind the feet of the swimmer in front of you. You can also get a less impressive draft by swimming on someone else's hip.

Another good question is whether this work-saving strategy

does you any good in the rest of the race. In September 2003, Delextrat et al attempted to answer this question in terms of the cycling leg of the race.[90] He had all of his study subjects wear wetsuits during a 750M swim, and then tested them for 15 minutes on a cycle ergometer. He then repeated this with a swimmer who was drafting. They found that there was a 7% decrease in heart rate while drafting versus not drafting, which was in line with previous studies. Also, lactate levels were 29% lower in the drafting trial. This is all well and good, and shows the effect of drafting on physiology. The interesting part was that they were able to show a 4.8% increase in cycling efficiency and a decrease in overall energy expenditure when biking after drafting versus not drafting on the swim.

Now we move onto the bike leg, where really significant gains can be made through drafting. The problem is that drafting is illegal except in ITU sanctioned races. However, should you find yourself in this situation; you ought to take advantage of the draft. There have been a number of studies showing this. Broker et al in 1999 described the power requirements at varying places in a pace line at 60 kph. This is a fair bit faster than the average ITU triathlon cycling leg, but will serve to make the point. If we consider the person at the front of the line maintaining 100% of the power required to hold 60kph, the 2nd man is only putting out 70.8%, the 3rd need only put out 64.1%, and the 4th 64%.[91]

If you choose to sit in the pack, you are best off a few racers back from the front to take maximal advantage of the draft. This might be a good strategy if you are a particularly fast runner. However, if you are a good cyclist and the pack seems to be watching one another rather than pushing the pace, you might be well advised to test the waters and put an attack in. If you get a minute or two on your competition, chances are that they might not be able to reel you in. Should you choose to do this, you must realize the effect of drafting on the subsequent run. As you might expect, it is beneficial. Hausswirth et al demonstrated that drafting on the cycling leg led to a 4.1% increase in running velocity afterwards.[92] Thus, your competition will be coming at you a little quicker than you might predict.

There is a fair amount of strategy outside the realm of drafting, which was well reviewed by David Swain at sportsci.org.[93] He makes a few important points which should influence not only your strategy, but your race selection. Earlier, we discussed the fact that power to weight ratio is important. We also know that surface area is important in terms of wind resistance (see chapter 10 for more on this). Specifically, mass and power increase with the 3rd power of height, whereas surface area increases only with the 2nd power. Thus, larger cyclists will do better in flat races, where the major opposition to speed is wind resistance because their power increases more quickly than their drag does.

In terms of hills, this relationship does not matter because race speeds are not fast enough for air resistance to be a factor. In those situations the racer with the highest power to weight ratio wins. Thus, the racer would be well advised to consider their size and power to weight ratio when deciding on what races to add to their program.

What about climbing technique? Swain addresses this as well with a computer simulation, which he published in the literature several years ago. On a hill that has equal uphill and downhill segments, we must remember that more time is spent climbing than is spent descending. Thus, there is a net loss of speed for the racer. The simulation indicated that small increases in power (on the order of 5%) on the uphill portion significantly reduces race time overall. Thus, the best strategy is to put in more effort on the climb and recover on the following downhill[93].

> **Small increases** in power going uphill significantly reduces race time overall.

My final comment on strategy regards drafting during the run: it seems to work to a limited extent. Astrand reports that there is significant benefit to sitting behind another runner. In 1971, Pugh studied the oxygen uptake of a runner out in the wind versus running approximately 1 meter behind another runner. He found there were significant gains to be made. During a 1500 meter race, a trailing runner can save up to 6% of the energy cost, or roughly 1 second per lap on the track.[94] This would be most important when running into a significant head wind or if dueling for the win at the finish line. If you have a finishing kick, you might be best advised to sit in, wait for the end, then sprint around and hope for the best.

Transitions

Although there is nothing scientific about the transition from one sport to the next, you will want to give this aspect of your race significant thought and preparation. It takes a major increase in fitness to knock a minute or two off of your 5k time or 800M swim; it takes just a little planning to save the same two minutes with an efficient switch from the swim to the bike or the bike to the run.

I'll give you a few suggestions, which are evident if you watch the tape of a few pro races and note how they orchestrate the transition. Practice getting out of your wetsuit: go down to the local lake or pool and work on getting out of the top as you are running through shallow water, then flopping on the ground and getting the bottom off. Practice getting into your bike shoes once they are already clipped to the pedals, rather than trying to slip and slide your way to the transition exit while running in them. Put elastic laces on your shoes so that you are not spending time tying them. You get the idea. Some experimentation will make a major difference in your times, and the improvement is very easily realized.

Fast transitions:

1. Practice getting out of your wetsuit.

2. Have your bike shoes clipped to the pedals and slip into them while riding away from T1.

3. Consider elastic laces for your running shoes.

CHAPTER 11

Aid By Technology

Swim Technology

The best aid to your swim time, after training, is likely a wetsuit. A recent study showed that swimming with a wetsuit reduced average heart rate by around 11%, and increased efficiency in a subsequent 10 minute bike trial by 12%.[95] It also speeds you up by decreasing the drag on your body. The wetsuit helps because the rubber has millions of air bubbles embedded in it, which helps you to float. This makes you more horizontal in the water, thus reducing the amount of frontal surface you present to the water as you move forward (figure 11.0). This of course means we must make the point that the wetsuit helps poor swimmers, who have poor body position, more than good swimmers. Whether or not you wear a wetsuit depends on one thing: do you spend more time getting out of it than you save by wearing it? In other words, you need to practice getting out of it quickly or you will blow all the time you saved. (This is less of an issue at Ironman, where there are wetsuit strippers at the swim exit to yank it off you). On the other hand, if your concern is simply finishing, then the wetsuit is

Without a wetsuit　　　With a wetsuit

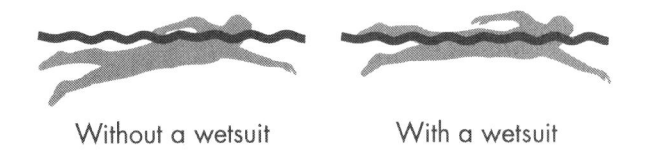

Figure 11.0　Body positioning without and with a wetsuit.

always an advantage because it saves you energy.

Next, if you are not going to wear a wetsuit, the question of shaving versus not shaving was answered by Sharp and Costill in 1989.[96] They tested two groups of swimmers twice during 90% effort swims of 365.8 meters. Half did not shave after the first test, half did. The results showed that the shaved group reduced their blood lactate by 25%, and increased their stroke length. In another group of swimmers, they also showed that shaving reduced the rate of slow down during a glide after pushing off of a wall. In other words, you'd be well advised to shave.

Finally, I am often asked about the high tech swimsuits often seen in Olympic competition. A study was published in June 2004 showing that at a speed of 2.2 meters/second, the shoulder-to-knee and shoulder to ankle suits produced 10-15% less drag than the other suits.[97] All designs were superior to simple briefs. Further, the suits did not cause a decrease in turn or dive speed. However, please note that no benefits were seen if the swimmers were going slower than 1.5 meters/second. Thus, if you swim the hundred in longer than 66 seconds, you can save your money.

Bike Technology: What Aero Can Do For You

Go by any bike race, triathlon, or bike shop, and you will see hundreds of examples of aerodynamic technology, the ostensible goal of which is to make you faster. If you read any of the trade magazines, you will see as many ads for the latest aero-wheels as you will for our aforementioned magic supplements. They both claim to make you faster, but as we saw, the supplements rarely meet the hype. We cannot make the same criticism of bike components: if they conform to certain well defined specifications, they will in fact make you at least somewhat faster based on the fact that they reduce aerodynamic drag on you or your bicycle. We will discuss the most important innovations in turn, in order to get you the most bang for your buck.

The most important aspect of your aerodynamic setup is your bike and your position on it. The reason is that your bike size, stem length and seat height are all-important in finding your "perfect fit." How well your machine fits you determine the position you are able to assume. Jim Martin (advisor to Team EDS and one of the minds behind Project 96, which was formed to design aerodynamic bikes for the 1996 Olympics) determined that roughly 85% of the aerodynamic drag of the rider/bicycle package is the result of pushing your body through the air.[98] If we can streamline the rider, we have gone a long way toward improving speed. A well positioned rider with a good aero position will beat the rider with all the aero goodies but an average or poor position every day of the week and twice on Sunday. You may have your heart set on that new $3000 time-trial bike with the aero frame and all the trimmings, but if it doesn't fit, you are wasting time, money, and training.

> **85% of drag is the result of pushing your body through the air.**

Now, the truth is that you can probably get a reasonable fit on just about any bicycle, provided you stick a long or short enough stem on it with an appropriate height seat post with appropriate set-back. However, this doesn't mean that any bike handles just like any other bike. The distribution of your weight over the wheels is determined by the geometry of the bike, how far you are hanging off the front, etcetera. This in turn determines how it will corner and the like. All of these factors will determine how fast you can go before we even start going into positioning or aerodynamics. The long and short of it is that we need a machine that fits you the best as a baseline to improve on.

Martin put together some pretty complex mathematical equations, which are beyond the scope of our discussion here. Essentially, given power out put of the rider, wind speed and direction, and the grade of the road, they can predict rider speed over a given course to within a percent or two. This was borne out by a paper by Martin et al in 1995.[99] What falls out of the wind tunnel data and math is the following. A 70 kg rider with a typical position on the aerobars generates about 8 lbs. of drag. With good positioning, that number can be reduced to 7, and with a truly excellent one, 6 lbs[98]. The question is, what does that mean to you and I out on the bike course of our local 40k time trial? A purely recreational cyclist at 8 lbs of drag, with a power output of 150 watts, would finish this course in around 77 minutes. The better position with 7 lbs. drag would reduce that time to 74 minutes. At 6 lbs drag, 70.5 minutes[98].

As you can see, there is significant time to be had without buying anything more expensive than a set of aerobars and maybe a new stem to put them in the right place under you. 7 minutes is roughly the difference between first and last place amongst elite racers in triathlon. It is worth taking some time to get the right fit.

An interesting thing that falls out of the math is that the slower you are, the more time you save by improving aerodynamics. This can be explained simply by the fact that the slower riders are out in the wind longer than the faster ones. But even a category one cyclist, with a power output of 350 watts, would save 5 minutes over the course of the above race.

What Goes into a Good fit

There are a couple of ways of looking at this. There is the most aerodynamic position you can possibly get into, there is the most powerful position you can be in, and then there is the most comfortable position we can get you into. The trick is finding a happy marriage between the three. If I position you and reduce your drag to 5 lbs, but you are twisted up like a pretzel and have to sit up halfway through the race, I didn't do you any good. Likewise, if I position you so that you look like a city bus going into the wind, you will very comfortably go very slowly. The first thing we will discuss is what seems to make a good aero position. Please note that these are general guidelines. You really need a wind tunnel to get it perfect, but unless you have five hundred bucks an hour and a bunch of scientists at your disposal, we might as well take the words of Dr. Martin and John Cobb, as they have spent hundreds of hours there.

If you have the time, inclination, a digital camera and/or video camera, and a stationary trainer, along with a desire to spend a lot of time tweaking, I feel you can probably get into the right ballpark. Do not delude yourself into thinking that this will be easy. You will be surprised at the difference in feel, comfort, and bike handling that results from what seems like insignificant changes in stem length or seat height. You can learn to tolerate and adapt to just about anything, but I feel that if you are planning on dropping a lot of money on a racing bike, it ought to fit you like a glove. The final adjustment may require a visit to a fitter, or a shop that does a good deal of fitting.

The benefit of seeing an experienced fitter is that he or she has set up literally hundreds of people, and very quickly picks up on fine points that someone with less experience might not. I have done a lot of bike fitting, but when I had issues with my own bike fit, I needed another set of eyes. As we said earlier regarding doctors, you can't diagnose or treat your own problems objectively. It was easy for my fitter to see that I was trying to ride in a position that was too aggressive, which I did not want to see for myself. Again, much like paying a doctor for their professional opinion, you are paying a good bike fitter for theirs. You will want to go with someone who is well recommended; who you believe has your best interests at heart, and is not necessarily trying to sell you the latest new gee-golly-whiz-bang accessory.

It is not my intention to promote or discount any particular fit system, as I do not have experience with all of them. In point of fact, we are all limited by economics and geography, so we tend to work with people who are in the neighborhood. You may not have a renowned fitter in your neighborhood. My point in writing this is to give you a general outline of some widely held principles, so that you can evaluate and decide on your own.

To answer a question I get often: I do not have a set fit system. I have some general guidelines which I have been able to take from many years of studies of anatomy and physiology, and I apply those basic principles of structure and function to the person I am working with. I will say that many times, when I look at riders who have been set up by another experienced fitter, I realize I would have done little different. I think for the most part, good fitters end up at the same destination; they just take different roads to get there.

What position is "Best"? (Or, Do I need a "Tri-Bike"?)
To some extent, the bike you buy is going to affect the position you ride in. The important question then becomes, "Is there any information that suggests one bike position is better than another?" Not surprisingly, there has been scientific study in this area.

In 1997, Gnehm et al looked at the influence of racing position on metabolic cost.[100] In other words, his group asked the question "Is one body position any more efficient than any other?" They tested cyclists while riding on the tops of their handlebars, riding on the drops, and riding on the aerobars. They found that as the riders assumed the more aero positions, their metabolic cost went up and their mechanical efficiency went down. The results indicate that switching from riding to upright to riding in the drops increases VO_2 by 1.5%, and by another 1.5% when moving from the drops to the aerobars. So, if you simply slap some aerobars on your road bike, you are putting yourself roughly at a 1.5-3% disadvantage, depending upon how you usually ride. However, this is well made up for by the amount of energy saved by being more aerodynamic.

Now, another study evaluated cardio-respiratory responses to change in seat tube angle. Was a more forward position better than a more rearward position? What they found was that as the seat tube angle moved from 69 degrees to 76 degrees, to 80 degrees and finally 90 degrees, there was a large detriment to VO_2 at 69 degrees, and all of the steeper angles fared similarly.[101] In this study, only the seat tube angle was changed. Thus, as the rider was moved forward on the bicycle, his hip angle opened up by a few degrees. Thus riding with the knees very close to the chest

(69 degrees) would seem to induce a physiologic change (recruitment of extra muscles, compression of blood vessels, etc) that causes an increase in energy expenditure.

Taken together, these results would seem to indicate that the best option is to ride a steep position bike if the rules allow it, to preserve the openness of the hip angle. Klippel and Heil have presented a model which showed that the optimal bicycle geometry is dependant upon the cyclist's usual preferred training geometry.[102] Again, invoking the principle of specificity, we would expect that the best results would be achieved with training specifically in the geometry we plan to race in. This is a problem if the athlete trains and races both on shallow angle road bikes and steep angled triathlon/time trial bikes. My advice would be the following: attempt to match your hip angles on both your road and triathlon bikes. This will at least ensure that some of your muscles are being trained and raced in the same orientation.

With those points out of way, let's get into the nitty-gritty of the wind tunnel. These seem to be some common factors which are important irrespective of absolute position on the bicycle. I would also ask for a bit of leeway here in terms of exact citations: this information comes from many disparate sources, often non-traditionally published sources including posts by the gurus of cycling aerodynamics on Internet chat boards. I have attempted to minimize the amount of information that comes directly from manufacturers, as they have a vested interest in convincing you to use their product.

The Horizontal Torso

The overwhelming message of all of the wind tunnel data seems to be that the most aero positions are the ones that limit how much of your frontal area is exposed to the wind.[103] Or rather, that the more frontal area, the more drag. When you sit more upright, the air streams into your chest. The lower you sit, the less of your chest is exposed to the wind, and the easier you cut through it. Thus, the first thing you want to get your torso as close to horizontal as is comfortably possible. In this way, it is really just the top surfaces of your shoulders and head that are facing the wind, as opposed to your head, neck, shoulders and chest.

The problem with this position is that your thighs will start to hit your chest when you lean that far down. Thus, as we stated above, you will need to move forward, either by moving your seat forward, or by riding a bike that has a steeper seat tube...in other words, one that moves the seat closer to the front of your bike. You will also need to lower your handlebars. This will allow you to increase the distance between your thighs and your chest to the distance they are when you are riding a standard road bike.

This is not absolutely necessary, of course, and in fact we determined above that the difference is on the order of 3% at most. Many of the riders in the Tour De France operate under rules that strictly limit how far forward they are allowed to sit, and I venture to say they are far faster than most triathletes will ever be. These riders generally do a couple of things, however. Firstly, they move their seats as far forward as the rules allow. Secondly, they sit on the very tip of their seats, which scoots them forward more, which is not terribly comfortable. Unless you ride in UCI sanctioned races, you don't need to resort to these measures, at least not today. However, rule changes are on the way, and in the next couple of years riders in US cycling races will need to conform to these regulations. Fortunately, USA Triathlon does not follow these rules, and you can ride practically any geometry you like (within reason).

The Narrow Elbows

Aerodynamic work by Cobb has indicated that the elbows do not need to be extremely narrow to realize benefits.[104] It seems that the only need to be narrow enough to block out your thighs/hips from the front, so that your thighs are in effect drafting behind your arms. Also, placing the hands closer together seems to work better than having them far apart, but this difference is debatable and is not as significant as the other factors we have discussed.

Knocking the Knees

Riding with your knees close to the top tube can make as much difference as a pair of aerodynamic wheels[98]. Once more, you are reducing the amount of your body surface area facing the wind, and preventing more air from entering the space between your legs, which already has a lot of air trying to squeeze through.

Equipment

Once you have realized your greatest gains through optimization of your position, it is time to start thinking about your equipment.

Wheels

According to Jim Martin[98], wheels account for 10% of the total drag on the bicycle system. So again, we have a situation where we can intervene to increase speed. Bar none, the fastest things you can put on your bike are disk wheels. The problem is that a disk wheel on the front of your bike is going to send you off into the trees when you are hit by a cross-wind. The other problem is that front disk wheels are illegal in most races, which rules them out anyway. However, you can almost always use them on the rear wheel (the notable exception being Ironman Hawaii), and there aren't many other aerodynamic additions you can make which will have as dramatic a result. John Cobb has reported that it takes roughly 35 watts to spin a 32 spoked wheel through the air at race speeds. It takes only 5-10 watts to spin a disk wheel, and perhaps 10-20 for a deep section aero or trispoke wheel[104].

If you don't think this is a significant difference, I have a simple experiment for you. Go down to the gym, get on the exercise bike, and start pedaling. Push the button that allows you to see your power output in watts, and set the resistance so that you are spinning your legs at a comfortable pace and your power output is, say, 200 watts. Do this for a few minutes, then decrease the resistance by 20-30 watts. What you are feeling is the difference between regular spoked wheels and the disk wheel. What this means is that you can go the same speed with less effort, or that you can go faster at the same effort. Either way, it is free speed (in terms of energy, not money!)

There are different types of disc wheels available: Lenticular and Flat. Lenticular means that the disc is lens shaped, i.e. curved on the sides, while the flat disks are flat sided. There has, in fact, been research to show that the lens shaped disc is slightly faster than the flat sided, but we are really splitting hairs and are not talking about more than a couple of seconds difference between them. These come at various price points, but rest assured that any disk wheel is a major upgrade. It is really a matter of how much you are willing to spend.

With regard to the deep section wheels, deeper is generally better in terms of aerodynamics, and this is agreed upon by the likes of Cobb and anyone else who has spent significant time in the wind tunnel. In fact, the only players who seem to dispute this fact are the companies who market solely "semi-deep" or shallow section wheel sets. There is some truth to the fact that bladed spokes, as well as reduced spoke count, will improve aerodynamics, however, the most important factor is always the rim depth. The fastest wheel seems to be the Hed3 (tri-spoke), which was originally developed by the DuPont corporation at considerable expense for use by the Olympic athletes. More money and brainpower went into this design than likely any other. However, faster is somewhat relative in this case as the choice between the Hed tri-spoke and a standard deep section rim of 40-60mm is likely a few seconds over 40k.

Run Technology

As we stated earlier in this manuscript, weight is extremely important in weight bearing exercise. It becomes even more important when the exercise involves hill climbing. In a running race, the heaviest thing on your person is likely your shoes. A paper by Holewijn et al in 1992 looked at energetic cost and stated that it is between 2 and 4 times more costly to wear heavy shoes than it was to add an additional kilogram to body weight.[105] Presumably, this results from the need to repeatedly lift the weight of the shoe with each step. Thus, we could argue that racing flats are faster than training shoes, provided that they are significantly lighter. I would caution you, however, to only use them while racing, and only if you are mechanically sound and injury free, and only for shorter races. Again, if you injure yourself using shoes that lack appropriate support, the amount of detraining you endure while recovering will easily outweigh the couple of extra seconds you gained while shedding a few ounces.

EPILOGUE

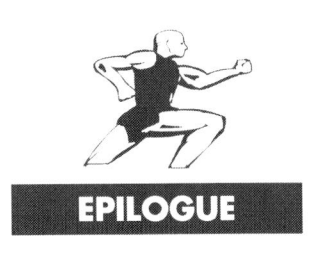

It is difficult to know when to end a work like this. There are thousands of volumes of information out there, coupled with innumerable people with extensive expertise. Rather than simply turn this into another physiology text, I will close with the suggestion that you continue your education in the science of exercise if it is of interest to you. You have the ability to improve your performance through the use of your mind, and I encourage you to do so. I have found that the benefit is twofold. Firstly, there is the tangible benefit of the reduction of your race times. Almost as important is the intangible benefit of knowing that your program is sound because you are educated, and having confidence that you will see commensurate results.

It is possible that you don't feel compelled to work through designing your own training programs. There is nothing wrong with this. However, in that instance I recommend that you employ a knowledgeable coach with background in exercise physiology, if you are interested in maximizing your performance. Don't accept cookie cutter training plans from a book, or from someone that does not know or understand your strengths, weaknesses, and goals as an athlete. If anything should be clear to you by reading this, it is that your best results will be realized by exercising with a purpose. Train smart.

Post Script

So What is a D.O., Anyway?

That is a good question, since we comprise less than 10 percent of the overall physician population in the United States. There are two degrees in the U.S. that can get you licensed as a physician: D.O. and M.D. The primary difference between these two degrees is that the D.O. (Doctor of Osteopathy), in addition to standard medical school, receives training in techniques of physical medicine, manipulation and therapy. After medical school, the D.O. might continue to offer those services if they are relevant to their field (for example, primary care or sports medicine), or they might not if they are practicing, for example, surgery or psychiatry. It should be noted that there are M.D. physicians out there that have taken courses in manipulative medicine who practice similarly, and even some who have additional degrees in physical therapy!

The bottom line is that both types of physicians are excellent. They practice equally in all scopes of medicine from obstetrics to neurosurgery. Their main difference (and there aren't many, nowadays) is that a D.O. who also practices physical manipulation and therapy (called Osteopathic Manipulative Therapy) may be somewhat better prepared to deal with your musculoskeletal complaints than a D.O. or M.D. who does not. You will likely get similar treatment from either, in the former case by hands-on therapy from your physician with the possible addition of a Physical Therapist, and in the latter cases by more PT and less direct physician participation. It is really a matter of preference on your part, but the difference might be worth investigating if you so choose.

Works Cited

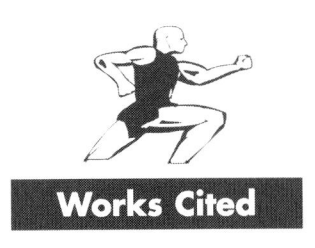

1. Wilmore JH and David L. Costill. Physiology of Sport and Exercise. Human Kinetics, Champaign, IL. 1999.

2. Wilmore JH and David L. Costill. Physiology of Sport and Exercise. Human Kinetics, Champaign, IL. 1999.

3. Coggan, AR. Training and racing using a power meter: an introduction. 2003.

4. Vachon et al. Validity of the heart rate deflection point as a predictor of lactate threshold during running. J. Appl. Physiol. 87(1):452-9. 1999.

5. Gaesser et al. Dissociation between VO2max and ventilatory threshold responses to endurance training. Eur J Appl Physiol Occup Physiol. 53(3):242-7. 1984.

6. Stoudemire et al. The validity of regulating blood lactate concentration during running by rating of perceived exertion. Med. Sci. Sports Exerc. 28(4) 490-95. 1996.

7. Tabata et al. Effects of moderate intensity and high intensity training on anerobic capacity and VO2max. Med. Sci. Sports Exerc. 28(10): 1327-30. 1997.

8. Billat et al. Intermittent runs at vVO2max enables subjects to remain at VO2max for a longer time than submaximal runs. Eur. J. Appl. Physiol. 81:188-96. 2000.

9. Carter et al. Effect of endurance training on oxygen uptake kinetics during treadmill running. J. Appl. Physiol. 89(5): 1744-1752. 2000.

10. Londeree BR. Effect of training on lactate/ventilatory thresholds: a meta analysis. Med. Sci. Sports Ex. 29:837-843. 1997.

11. Rhea et al. A meta-analysis to determine the dose response for strength development. Med. Sci. Sports Exerc. 35(3): 456–64. 2003.

12. Demarle et el. Whichever the initial training status, any increase in velocity at lactate threshold appears as a major factor in improved time to exhaustion at the very same severe velocity after training. Arch. Physiol. Biochem. 111(2): 167-76. 2003.

13. Coggan, AR. Training and racing using a power meter: an introduction. 2003.

14. Wilmore JH and David L. Costill. Physiology of Sport and Exercise. Human

Kinetics, Champaign, IL. 1999.

15. Wilmore JH and David L. Costill. Physiology of Sport and Exercise. Human Kinetics, Champaign, IL. 1999.

16. Wilmore JH and David L. Costill. Physiology of Sport and Exercise. Human Kinetics, Champaign, IL. 1999.

17. Billat et al. Physical and training characteristics of top class marathon runners. Med. Sci. Sports Exerc. 33(12): 2089-97. 2001.

18. Coyle e t al. Determinants of endurance in well-trained cyclists. J. Appl. Physiol. 64(6):2622-2630. 1988.

19. Hill D. and Amy Rowell. Responses to exercise at the velocity associated with VO2max. Med. Sci. Sports Exerc. 29(1):113-6. 1997.

20. Billat et al. Training and bioenergetic characteristics in elite male and female Kenyan runners. Med. Sci. Sports Exerc. 35(2): 297-4. 2003.

21. Lucia et al. Kinetics of vo2 in professional cyclists. Med. Sci. Sports Exerc. 34(2): 320-5, 2002.

22. Lucia et al. Physiology of professional road cycling. Sports Med. 31: 325-37. 2001.

23. Gaesser et al. The slow component of oxygen uptake kinetics in humans. Ex. Sport Sci. Rev. 24:35-50. Williams and Wilkins. 1996.

24. Astrand et al. Textbook of Work Physiology: Physiologic Bases of Exercise. 4th ed. Human Kinetics, Champaign, IL. 2004.

25. Astrand et al. Textbook of Work Physiology: Physiologic Bases of Exercise. 4th ed. Human Kinetics, Champaign, IL. 2004.

26. Noakes, Timothy. Commentary in Med. Sci. Sports Exerc. 35(2). 2003.

27. Coyle et al. Physiological and biomechanical factors associated with elite endurance cycling performance. Med. Sci. Sports Exerc. 23(1):93-107. 1991.

28. Zoldaz et al. VO2/Power output relationship and the slow component of oxygen uptake kinetics during cycling at different pedaling rates: relationship to venous lactate accumulation and blood acid-base balance. Physiol. Res. 47: 427-438. 1998.

29. Astrand et al. Textbook of Work Physiology: Physiologic Bases of Exercise. 4th ed. Human Kinetics, Champaign, IL. 2004.

30. Gaskill et al. Responses to training in cross-country skiers. Med. Sci. Sports Exerc. 31(8): 1211-7. 1999.

31. Magel at al. Specificity of swim training on maximum oxygen uptake. J. Appl. Physiol. 38(1)151-5. 1975.

32. Coyle et al. Physiological and biomechanical factors associated with elite endurance cycling performance. Med. Sci. Sports Exerc. 23(1):93-107. 1991.

33. Wilmore JH and David L. Costill. Physiology of Sport and Exercise. Human Kinetics, Champaign, IL. 1999.

34. Marcinik et al. Effect of strength training on lactate threshold and endurance performance. Med. Sci. Sports Exerc. 23(6) 739-43. 1991.

35. McCartney et al. Usefulness of weightlifting training in improving strength and maximal power output in coronary artery disease. Am. J. Card. 67(11):939-45. 1991.

36. Hickson et al. Potential for strength and endurance training to amplify endurance performance. J. Appl. Phys. 65(5):2285-90. 1988.

37. Bastiaans JJ et al. The effects of replacing a portion of endurance training by explosive strength training on performance in trained cyclists. Eur J. Appl. Physiol. 86(1):79-84. 2001.

38. Tanaka et al. Dry-land resistance training for competitive swimming. Med. Sci. Sports Exerc. 25:952-9. 1993.

39. Hawley J. Http:// www.sportsci.org/news/traingain/resistance.html. Accessed March 2004

40. Astrand et al. Textbook of Work Physiology: Physiologic Bases of Exercise. 4th ed. Human Kinetics, Champaign, IL. 2004.

41. Coyle et al. Time course of loss of adaptations after stopping prolonged intense endurance training. J. Appl. Phys. 57(6) 1857-64. 1984.

42. Mujika I and S Padilla. Detraining: Loss of training induced physiological and performance adaptations. Part II: Long term insufficient training stimulus. Sports Med. 30(3):145-54. 2000.

43. Coyle et al. Effect of detraining on cardiovascular responses to exercise: role of blood volume. J. Appl. Phys. 60(1):95-9. 1986.

44. Astrand et al. Textbook of Work Physiology: Physiologic Bases of Exercise. 4th ed. Human Kinetics, Champaign, IL. 2004.

45. Ingjer, F. Maximal oxygen uptake as a predictor of performance ability in women and men elite cross-country skiers. Scand. J. Med. Sci. Sports 1:25-30. 1991.

46. Noakes TD. The Lore of Running. 4th edition. Human Kinetics, Champaign, IL. 2002.

47. Daniels J. Daniels' Runnning Formula. Human Kinetics, Champaign, IL. 1998.

48. Busso, T. Variable dose-response relationship between exercise training and performance. Med. Sci. Sports Exerc. 35(7) 1188-1195. 2003.

49. Bannister et al. A systems model of training for athletic performance. Aust. J. Sports Med. 7:57-61. 1975.

50. Morton et al. Modeling human performance in running. J. Appl. Physiol. 69:1171-7. 1990

51. Acevedo, EO and A H Goldfarb. Increased training intensity effects on plasma lactate, ventilatory threshold, and endurance. Med. Sci. Sports Exerc. 21:563-568, 1989.

52. Burke et al. Carbohydrate intake during prolonged cycling minimizes effect of glycemic index of preexercise meal. J. Appl. Physiol. 85(6): 2220-6. 1998.

53. Roy L. P. G. et al. High Oxidation Rates from combined carbohydrates ingested during exercise. Med. Sci. Sports Exerc. 36(9): 1551-8. 2004.

54. Astrand et al. Textbook of Work Physiology: Physiologic Bases of Exercise. 4th ed. Human Kinetics, Champaign, IL. 2004.

55. Zawadzki et al. Carbohydrate –protein complex increases the rate of muscle glycogen storage after exercise. J. Appl. Phys. 72(5): 1854-9. 1992.

56. Tarnopolski et al. Postexercise protein-carbohydrate and carbohydrate supplements increase muscle glycogen in men and women. J. Appl. Phys. 83(6): 1877-3. 1997.

57. Jentjens et al. Addition of protein and amino acids to carbohydrates does not enhance postexercise muscle glycogen synthesis. J. Appl. Physiol. 91(2): 839-46. 2001.

58. Noakes TD. Hyponatremia in distance runners: fluid and sodium balance during exercise. Curr. Sports Med. Rep. 4:197-207. 2002.

59. Speedy et al. Oral salt supplementation during ultradistance exercise. Clin. J. Sports Med. 12(5): 279-84. 2002.

60. Ariel et al. Effect of anabolic steroids on reflex components. J. Appl. Physiol. 32(6):795-7. 1972.

61. Carey et al. Effects of fat adaptation and carbohydrate restoration on prolonged endurance exercise. J. Appl. Physiol. 91:115-22. 2001.

62. Jeukendrup et al. Oxidation of carbohydrate feedings during prolonged exercise: cur-

rent thoughts, guidelines and directions for future research. Sports Med. 29: 407-24. 2000.

63. Kovacs et al. Effect of caffeinated drinks on substrate metabolism, caffeine excretion, and performance. J. Appl. Physiol. 85(2):709-15. 1998.

64. Bell DG and TM McLellan. Exercise endurance 1, 3, and 6h after caffeine ingestion in caffeine users and nonusers. J. Appl. Physiol. 93:1227-34. 2002.

65. Van Nieuwenhoven et al. Gastrointestinal function during exercise: comparison of water, sports drink, and sports drink with caffeine. J. Appl. Physiol. 89:1079-85. 2000.

66. Angus et al. Effect of carbohydrate or carbohydrate plus medium chain triglyceride ingestion on cycling time trial performance. J. Appl. Physiol. 88:113-119. 2000.

67. De La Vieja et al. Creatine and creatine metabolism. Physio. Reviews 80(3): 1107-1213 (2000).

68. Hultman et al. Muscle creatine loading in men. J. Appl. Physiol. 81(1): 232-7. 1996.

69. Smith et al. Creatine supplementation and age influence muscle metabolism during exercise. J. Appl. Physiol. 85: 1349-56. 1998.

70. Harris et al. The effect of oral creatine supplementation on running performance during maximal short term exercise. J. Appl. Physiol. 467:74. 1993.

71. Earnest et al. Effects of a commercial herbal based formula on exercise performance in cyclists. Med. Sci. Sports Exerc. 36(3): 504-509. 2004.

72. Lage et al. Cyclist's doping associated with cerebral sinus thrombosis. Neurology. 58(4). 665. 2001.

73. Jacobs et al. Effects of Ephedrine, Caffeine, and Their Combination on Muscular Endurance. Med. Sci. Sports Exerc. 35(6): 987–94. 2003.

74. Bell et al. Effect of ingesting caffeine and ephedrine on 10-km run performance. Med. Sci. Sports Exerc. 34(2): 344–9. 2002.

75. Neary et al. The effects of a reduced exercise duration taper program on performance and muscle enzymes of endurance cyclists. Eur. J. Appl. Physiol. Occup. Physiol. 65(1):30-6. 1995.

76. Neary et al. Effects of taper on endurance cycling capacity and single muscle fiber properties. Med. Sci. Sports Exerc. 35(11):1875-81. 2003.

77. Trappe et al. Effect of swim taper on whole muscle and single muscle fiber contractile properties. Med. Sci. Sports Exerc. 32(12):48-56. 2000.

78. Mujika et al. Physiological responses to a 6-d taper in middle-distance runners: influence of training intensity and volume. Med. Sci. Sports Exerc. 32(2):511-7. 2000.

79. Houmard et al. The effects of taper on performance in distance runners. Med. Sci. Sports Exerc. 26(5):624-31. 1994.

80. Mujika and Padilla. Scientific bases for precompetition tapering strategies. Med. Sci. Sports Exerc. 35(7):1182-7. 2003.

81. Banister et al. Training theory and taper: validation in triathlon athletes. Eur. J Appl. Physiol. Occup Physiol. 79(2):182-91. 1999.

82. Kenitzer. Optimal taper period in female swimmers. J. Swimming Res. 13:31-36. 1998.

83. Kubukeli and T.D. Noakes. Training techniques to improve endurance exercise performance. Sports Med. 32:489-509. 2002.

84. Houmard et al. The Effect of warm up on responses to intense exercise. Int. J. Sports Med. 12(5):480-3. 1991.

85. Thacker et al. The impact of stretching on sports injury risk: a systematic review of the literature. Med. Sci. Sports Exerc. 36(3) 371-378. 2004.

86. Moller et al. Duration of stretching effect on range of motion in lower extremities. Arch PM&R 66:171-5. 1985.

87. Zebas et al. Retention of flexibility in selected joints after cessation of stretching exercise program. Ex. Phys: Current selected research. 181-91. 1985.

88. Dengel et al. Determinants of success during triathlon competition. Res. Q. Ex. Sp. 60:234-238. 1989.

89. Chatard JC et al. Performance and drag during drafting swimming in highly trained triathletes. Med. Sci. Sports. Exerc. 30:1276-1280. 1998.

90. Dextrelat et al. Drafting during swimming improves efficiency during subsequent cycling. Med. Sci. Sports Exerc. 35(9): 1612-9. 2000.

91. Broker et al. Racing cyclist power requirements in the 4000m individual and team pursuits. Med. Sci. Sports Exerc. 31(11). 1999.

92. Hausswirth et al. Effect of cycling alone or in a sheltered position on subsequent running performance during a triathlon. Med Sci. Sports Exerc. 31:599-604. 1999.

93. Swain et al. Cycling Uphill and Downhill. http://www.sportsci.org. Accessed Spring 2004.

94. Astrand et al. Textbook of Work Physiology: Physiologic Bases of Exercise. 4th ed. Human Kinetics, Champaign, IL. 2004.

95. Delextrat et al. Effects of swimming with a wet suit on energy expenditure during subsequent cycling. Can. J. Appl. Phys. 28(3):356-69. 2003.

96. Sharp et al. Influence of body hair removal on physiological responses during breaststroke swimming. Med. Sci. Sports Exerc. 21(5):576-80. 1989.

97. Mollendorf et al. Effect of swim suit design on passive drag. Med. Sci. Sports Exerc. 36(6): 1029-35. 2004.

98. Martin J. Http://www.cervelo.com/tech/articles/article5.html. Accessed Spring 2004.

99. Martin et al. Validation of a Mathematical Model for Road Cycling Power. J. Appl. Biomech. 14: 276-291. 1998.

100. Gnehm et al. Influence of different racing positions on metabolic costs in elite cyclists. Med. Sci. Sports Exerc. 29(6): 818-23. 1997.

101. Heil et al. Cardiorespiratory responses to seat tube variation during steady state cycling. Med. Sci. Sports Exerc. 27:730-5. 1995.

102. Klippel and DP Heil. A simulation for determining the optimal bicycle geometry for a flat time trial. Med. Sci. Sports Exerc. 34(5):S25

103. Bassett et al. Comparing cycling world hour records. 1967-1996: modeling with empirical data. Med. Sci. Sports Exerc. 31(11)1665-76. 1999.

104. Cobb J. Http://www.bicyclesports.com. Accessed Fall 2002.

105. Holewijn et al. Physiological strain due to load carrying in heavy footwear. Eur. J. Appl. Physiol. Occup. Physiol. 65(2):129-34. 1992.

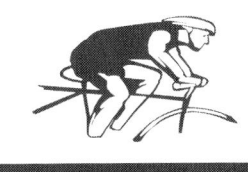

ABOUT THE AUTHOR

Dr. Skiba completed his undergraduate training in biology at Siena College, in Loudonville, NY. From there, he went on to finish a master's degree in Microbiology and Molecular Genetics at The University of Medicine and Dentistry of NJ- New Jersey Medial School. Dr. Skiba completed medical school at KCOM, in Kirksville, MO in June of 2003, and finished an internship in Internal Medicine at Lutheran General Hospital (Park Ridge, IL) in June 2004. He is currently a resident at The National Rehabilitation Hospital/Georgetown University in Washington D.C., where he is training in Physical Medicine and Rehabilitation. Dr. Skiba has been racing competitively in triathlon for four years, and in cycling for 2 years. He has been swimming, biking, skiing, hiking, surfing and running for enjoyment and health for over 20 years.

In a continuing effort to help educate and train triathletes and other endurance enthusiasts, Dr. Skiba founded PhysFarm.com, a coaching service for multisport athletes, where he personally manages and advises all clients.

PhysFarm
training smart

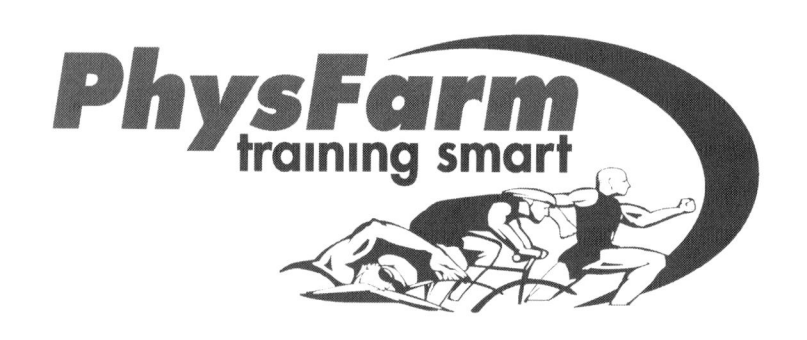

▶ Interested in learning more?

▶ Interested in having Dr. Skiba as your personal coach?

Log onto www.PhysFarm.com
for more information, training tips,
and ways to make scientific principles
part of your training regimen.

www.PhysFarm.com